Praise for *Living an Orgasmic Life*

"Xanet Pailet's book offers a modern, refreshing insight into what all women should become aware of: that they are made for love. And that the art and cultivation of pleasure is the language of love. And that if they don't learn it and take the responsibility to teach it to their partners, the consciousness of the world will remain stagnant. *Living an Orgasmic Life* teaches us to become aware in love and to channel pleasure as a means of conscious awakening. There is no better mission. And this book will show you the way."

—Margot Anand, the world's leading authority on Tantra, and international bestselling author of *The Art of Sexual Ecstasy, The Art of Everyday Ecstasy*, and *Love, Sex and Awakening*

"Through her own sexual healing journey and those of others, author and intimacy coach Xanet Pailet takes us back to a place where we can all develop the courage to reclaim our sexual desires. *Living an Orgasmic Life* is bound to become a go-to book for therapists, for healers, and for all of us."

—Louann Brizendine, MD, *New York Times* bestselling author of *The Female Brain* and *The Male Brain*

"A woman who's been there—out of touch with her own capacity for erotic connection and pleasure—and healed herself, tackles all the stumbling blocks for other people's inability to touch this deep source of joy. Fraught social messages, shame, and trauma impact so many of us, but as Xanet Pailet shows, there IS a path out of that thicket and into intimacy, deep sexual pleasure, and a newly-awakened body. Take this journey with her and be amazed at the destination."

—Carol Queen PhD, Staff Sexologist, Good Vibrations

"Xanet is a wise guide that you can trust to lead you to the pleasurable path of erotic empowerment. She's been there herself and offers you a practical map that you can follow to get to the land of loving yourself, shame-free sex, and expanded outrageous orgasms! You deserve to feel this fantastic!"
—Sheri Winston, CNM, RN, LMT, Wholistic Sexuality Teacher, award-winning author of *Women's Anatomy of Arousal* and *Succulent SexCraft*

"The parts of this book that touched me deeply, and what will reach out and touch the hearts of so many women, are the moments when Xanet shares her personal journey of growth and transformation. Her vulnerability, raw honesty, and deep desire to learn and teach what is possible for women in the erotic realm touches on the hopes and insecurities we all have. By sharing those parts that we feel we are supposed to hide, she fearlessly invites women to know and accept themselves fully so they can claim their birthright of pleasure."
—Celeste Hirschman, MA, cofounder Somatica Institute, author of *Cockfidence* and *Making Love Real*

"Can you imagine your life and loving to be abundant with creative energy, confidence, inner freedom, and good feelings about yourself, a state of being where old wounding no longer rules you and your sexual experience? This book contains the keys to unlock your sexual potential, open yourself to more bliss, and let go of what no longer serves you. Xanet's practices and real-life stories will help you to heal any sexual wounds and move beyond shame into a powerful connection with yourself, transforming your entire life into an everyday orgasmic experience. While presenting a myriad of expertise and information, its easy-to-read style captivates the heart and soul and gently invites the reader to a journey of transformation and healing. A must-read for anyone willing to expand their horizon and live more orgasmically every day."

—Lokita Carter, founder of Ecstatic Living Institute, creator of bestselling video programs on Tantra and Chakra Wisdom Meditation

"This book is an excellent blend of personal stories, solid research, useful ideas, and supportive suggestions. If you're struggling to figure out how to connect to your pleasure, make sex exciting, and deepen your relationship, there's plenty of great information here for you and your partner."

—Charlie Glickman, PhD, Sex and Relationship coach, author of *The Ultimate Guide to Prostate Pleasure*, www.makesexeasy.com

"Unabashed reality, heartfelt empathy, keen expertise—all three combine in this breakthrough work by Xanet Pailet. As a Sexual Abuse Recovery Coach, I am always on the lookout for quality resources that will support my clients in finding their way to freedom in this area of their lives, and *Living an Orgasmic Life* is now at the top of my reading list for survivors who want to reclaim their sexuality."

—Rachel Grant, author of *Beyond Surviving: The Final Stages in Recovery from Sexual Abuse* and the *Beyond Surviving* podcast

"Xanet Pailet has written one of the most sex-positive books on women's sexuality in *Living an Orgasmic Life: Heal Yourself and Awaken your Pleasure*. This book will open hearts and minds and change lives! I highly recommend this as a must-read for all my colleagues & clients!"

—Rev. Michele Clarkson MSW, LCSW, AASECT Certified Diplomate Sex Therapist with thirty-nine years of experience in the field of sexology

Living an Orgasmic Life is dedicated to the teachers, mentors, and healers who have been such an integral part of my journey over the past decade. There are too many of them to list, but they know exactly who they are. Without their support, friendship, wisdom, and healing touch, my personal transformation, growth and sexual awakening would not have been possible. Words are insufficient to express my gratitude.

Living
an
Orgasmic
Life

For permission requests, please contact the publisher at:

Mango Publishing Group
2850 Douglas Road, 3rd Floor
Coral Gables, FL 33134 U.S.A.
info@mango.bz

For special orders, quantity sales, course adoptions and corporate sales, please email the publisher at sales@mango.bz. For trade and wholesale sales, please contact Ingram Publisher Services at:
customer.service@ingramcontent.com or +1.800.509.4887.

Living an Orgasmic Life: Heal Yourself and Awaken Your Pleasure

Library of Congress Cataloging
ISBN: (p) 978-1-63353-826-9, (e) 978-1-63353-827-6
Library of Congress Control Number: 2018944499
BISAC - HEA042000 — HEALTH & FITNESS / Sexuality

Disclaimer

This book is partially a memoir in which I have tried to recreate events, locales, and conversations from my memory. However, to protect people's privacy and anonymity, I have changed many identifying characteristics and details, such as names, places, and occupations. Individuals named in client stories are composite characters, gleaned from the hundreds of women and men who I have worked with.

This book is not intended as a substitute for the medical advice of physicians. The reader should regularly consult a health care provider in matters relating to his/her health and particularly with respect to any symptoms that may require diagnosis or medical attention.

Living an Orgasmic Life

HEAL YOURSELF AND AWAKEN YOUR PLEASURE

Xanet Pailet

Mango Publishing
CORAL GABLES, FL

CONTENTS

PART ONE

*Healing Yourself from Shame, Sexual Abuse,
and Physical Trauma*

PART TWO

Awakening Your Pleasure

Foreword

I was sitting alone on a break during the first week of our Somatica® Sex and Intimacy training program, putting out fires in my office and completely absorbed on my laptop. A woman came up to me and said, "Oh my God, you're Emily Morse. I have your Kegel app on my phone, and I recommend it to all my Holistic Pelvic Care clients. I am so excited to meet you!"

That afternoon, Xanet and I spent an hour talking about Holistic Pelvic Care. I quickly realized that this woman had a depth of knowledge, skills, and life experience about sexual healing and awakening that set her apart from many sex educators, coaches, and experts. After all, having lived in a sexless marriage for twenty-five years gives her a lot of street cred! Although relatively new to the field, Xanet is the real deal, and this book will prove it to you.

When I first read *Living an Orgasmic Life* in preparation for a *Sex with Emily* podcast with Xanet, I was surprised by how much I related to her personal story. Like Xanet, I grew up very disconnected from my body and sexuality. For many years, it was hard for me to experience pleasure and orgasms. I also struggled with intimacy and not having a good role model for what a healthy relationship should look like.

Feeling confused around sexuality is a state of mind I can relate to because I hear it all the time from my listeners. So many women struggle with sexless marriages, painful intercourse, inability to experience orgasm, and low libido. Not only does Xanet address all these issues in this book, but she provides a vast array of exercises and tools to help women find or reclaim their pleasure.

What I love the most about this book is the way in which Xanet masterfully weaves in her own story in such a vulnerable way.

She makes it completely relatable to every woman's experience and provides all of us a path forward to living an orgasmic life.

While there are many words of wisdom in this book, I want to leave you with this concept: Xanet talks about a woman's pelvic bowl (uterus, ovaries, vagina) as her second heart and second brain—the source of tremendous love and wisdom and the gateway to orgasmic life energy. *Living an Orgasmic Life* is born from this place of birth and rebirth, and I can already tell how profoundly this book will impact women and help us reconnect our sexuality to our emotions, body, and our pleasure. I am honored and delighted to be part of this book's orgasmic birth and to call Xanet a colleague and a friend.

DR. EMILY MORSE
Founder & Host of *Sex with Emily*

Introduction

The concept of an "orgasmic life" first appeared on the vision board I created five years ago when I started my business The Power of Pleasure after having just left a two decades long sexless marriage. To me, living an orgasmic life means that you are living a life that flows easily, without struggle, just like how an orgasm happens. What I learned on my journey of sexual healing and awakening is that sexuality is at the core of our being. It is powerful beyond words. Not only can it help us achieve a state of sexual bliss, but it can also alter the course of our entire life. Dynamic personal growth and transformation are available when a woman fully connects with her sexuality and orgasmic potential. When this happens, she will inevitably experience a flood of new life force energy and a surge of creativity. The result is typically a profound shift in her intimate life that ripples out into every part of her world.

In the pages that follow, I will share my story and the stories of other women and men who have made this surprising transformation. Read with an open heart, and you will begin to feel the vital flame of your sexuality begin to flicker. In each chapter, I will share essential lessons that can take your sex life from ho-hum or nonexistent to fulfilling on every level.

You will learn a practical approach that is simple, but not always easy. Through a process of inquiry and self-reflection, coupled with self-directed activities, you will discover:

- The many factors that cause women to shut down their sexuality
- Why it's so hard to talk about sex in a world where everything is about sex

- The number one reason women lose their desire for sex and what to do about it
- How sexual trauma can occur and how to heal it
- Your sexual blueprint: what it is and how to read it
- How attachment theory relates to your intimate life
- What the journey to sexual healing looks like
- How to find your path to pleasure
- Awakening your body through somatic and hands-on healing
- How to reignite your libido
- The truth about your pleasure potential
- What you can do to start living an orgasmic life in the bedroom and beyond

If I could transform my sex life at the age of fifty, I know for certain that you can as well, whether you are twenty-five or sixty-five. If you feel broken or disconnected from your sexual self, find yourself avoiding lovemaking, or can't sustain intimacy, this book will help you reclaim your sexuality and move toward living an orgasmic life. Welcome to the journey.

A Note about Terminology

For many women, what we call our sexual body parts is a charged subject. I recently had a woman walk out of one of my classes when I used the word "pussy." And while Donald Trump's sadly derisive use of the term during his 2016 presidential campaign made "pussy" a household word, it still makes many women uncomfortable. There are many words for vagina and penis from which to choose, and what is offensive to one woman may be endearing to another. I use words for sexual body parts interchangeably to help you see that a word is just a word. It's the connotation, belief system, and socialization that make words feel charged.

Here are the words for female and male genitalia I will use in this book:

- Vagina/Vulva
- Penis
- Pussy
- Cock
- Yoni
- Lingam

I encourage you to add to this list all the names you've heard, read, or used for vaginas and penises, including nicknames that you may have for your own, or your partner's, body parts. Then pick the ones that you like and start using them.

For My LGBTQ Friends

The nature of this book that recounts my own heteronormative relationships, as well as client case studies involving my client population, requires me to delve into the differences between cisgender men and women when it comes to intimacy and sexuality. I have tried to use gender-neutral terms wherever possible (e.g., "partner" rather than "wife/husband" or "boyfriend/girlfriend"). I hope that you will find much of the information in this book useful in examining your own relationships and sexuality regardless of the genders of the subjects.

PART ONE

.

Healing Yourself from Shame, Sexual Abuse, and Physical Trauma

Chapter 1

. . . .

ONE NIGHT CAN CHANGE YOUR LIFE

. . . .

At thirty-five years of age, I absolutely HATED sex. Everything about it was painful. Intercourse just plain hurt, and I'd landed in the doctor's office with female problems more times than I could count. Just thinking about sex was stressful. Talking about it was impossible. So, like many couples, my husband and I simply stopped having sex. If you had told me that I'd be having multiple orgasms, ejaculating, and riding hour-long waves of orgasmic pleasure in my fifties, I would have said, "You must be on drugs."

How does a woman who has lost all interest in sex and whose libido has been in a decades long slumber wake up to discover the delights of lovemaking, reclaim her sexuality, and begin to live an orgasmic life? It all started from a chance encounter on OK Cupid, an online dating site, where I met Eric, also known as "Tantra Man." Eric offered me an experience that changed the course of my life.

It was a hot summer night in Midtown Manhattan. When Eric welcomed me into his apartment, I smiled, breathing in the sweet smell of rosehips. He'd invited me over for a relaxed Sunday evening, promising a big surprise. He was an excellent cook and had made us dinner a couple times before, so I assumed the surprise was a special menu. Over the previous three days, I'd been musing about what might be in store. But he wasn't wearing his chef apron and designer jeans per usual. In fact, his attire was downright unusual: he was wearing nothing but a sarong, a body length multicolored scarf, tied around his waist. I was startled and a wee bit tongue-tied at first—I'd never seen anyone wear a sarong in New York—but managed to untie my tongue and ask, with just a hint of sarcasm, "So is that my surprise? We're going to Maui?"

He smiled, said, "Nooooooo…" and with a sweep of his arm, led me into the apartment, which was rather warm. I decided he must have chosen the sarong due to the heat and felt myself relax.

He directed me toward his beautiful leather sofa and I sat down. He placed a lovely tray of cheese, nuts, crudités, and crackers on the coffee table, along with an expensive bottle of red wine.

Hmmm…I thought. This, too, was a break from his usual behavior. He'd never served appetizers before. What in the world did he have in mind?

I'd met Eric several months earlier on OKCupid. When we first crossed paths, he was recently separated from his wife of many years. I found him to be incredibly needy, even clingy, and sexually aggressive in a way that really turned me off. Our relationship, such as it was, had been rather rocky. We'd broken up a couple of times over the first few months. He really hadn't a clue how to treat a woman, but he was extremely smart, interesting to talk to, and a successful businessman. We were so well-matched intellectually that I stayed in the game. Not in a gazillion years would I have guessed he'd be the man to change the game for me entirely.

Eric sat down on the couch a good foot and a half away from me. I was thankful for the space and once again noted this break from his usual behavior. In fact, he was displaying none of his typical neediness, which gave me a chance to feel a desire for closeness I'd never felt around him before.

He spread some soft goat cheese on a cracker and handed it to me. "Please have some."

I accepted and looked into his eyes. But I couldn't find the words to wonder aloud about the big surprise so I simply said, "Thank you." I was completely certain that he'd read the quizzical look on my face.

He smiled, moved about two inches closer to me on the couch, reached for some cashews, and turned his body to face me directly.

"I suppose you're wondering what's going on," he said. "Well, I spent the last two days in a workshop with a Tantra master."

I didn't have a frame of reference for a Tantra master, so I just nodded and waited for him to say more.

As he began to share his experience, I noticed that his demeanor was completely different than how I'd experienced him before. He was confident, kind, and loving, and his passion for this Tantra thing was so intoxicating that I barely heard a word he said. Nonetheless, as he continued to speak, I found myself leaning in, hoping to understand what he was saying.

"The really intriguing thing about Tantra," he said, "is the focus on worshipping the Goddess."

Again, I didn't have a frame of reference, other than the small big-bellied figurines I'd seen in a book about ancient matriarchal societies.

He moved back a little away from me and seemed to be taking my temperature on this idea, then said, "I was thinking we could dedicate this evening to Goddess worship."

Unsure of the meaning of this proposal, I said, "I'm not sure what you mean. Goddess worship?"

He explained that the workshop with the Tantra master had opened his eyes to a whole new world, a world he wanted to share with me...if I was willing. He described it as a world that would involve all of my senses, a world in which I would be the focus of his attention, a world where he would put his sexual desire aside and focus solely on my pleasure. "I simply want to worship you as the embodiment of the Goddess."

I stammered. Looked around the room for a place to hide. Battled my urge to race out the door and finally convinced myself that it couldn't hurt. I could always get up and leave if this Goddess worship thing turned into yet another failed romantic attempt. "I suppose," I said. "What do you want me to do?"

He smiled, picked up his iPad, and put on what he called his new "Tantra playlist." Then for the first time since I'd stepped through the door, he moved close, touched my knee and said, "You just sit there and enjoy the music. Have some cheese and nuts. I'm going to draw you a bath."

That first night of Goddess worship was one of the most amazing experiences of my life. I literally just lay on his bed and allowed myself to be pleasured with no expectations. I did not have crazy, screaming orgasms (those came later), but I did experience my body in a way I never had before. I didn't know I was capable of experiencing such an immense amount of pleasure. And the connection I felt to my sexuality was completely new to me.

That night was the beginning of a wondrous journey. I had a long road ahead of me, but that night lit a flame in my belly and gave me a mountain of hope. I did not have to be a broken woman forever.

Chapter 2

. . . .

LIVING A LIFE OF LIES

. . . .

What if I told you that, no matter your age, the best sex of your life is ahead of you? How would your life be different if you started having the most amazing sex of your life in the months and years ahead? I'm talking about mind-blowing, "Oh my God! —What the f*** was that!?" kind of sex. You can have orgasms that make you think you have died and gone to heaven; orgasms that rock your entire body; orgasms you feel from the tips of your toes to the top of your head; orgasms that last not just for minutes, but for hours; orgasms that make you scream and moan, and that take you out of your body into blissful dimensions previously unknown. This is the potential of your sexuality.

With extended orgasm, your biochemistry changes completely; it's like natural LSD.

Imagine feeling more pleasure in your body than you thought possible. How would it feel to be so sexually awake and alive that you can completely surrender to sensation and pleasure? This is my wish for you—to live an orgasmic life.

Appearances Can Be Deceiving

If you'd known me when I was forty years old, it's quite likely you would have thought that I was already living an orgasmic life. I'd turned my background in health care law into a very successful health care consulting business in New York City. I lived in a gorgeous apartment on the Upper West Side with my husband of twenty years and my two amazing boys. I oversaw a complete gutting and renovation of our New York apartment, personally selecting every piece of wood, granite, stone, and platinum. I was certain we would live there for the rest of our lives and that one of our boys would inherit the place. I was living THE life, with all the material trappings that went along with it. My kids went to the best schools in the city. We frequented the finest restaurants, took amazing vacations, and attended premiere Broadway openings and events. And yet I knew deep inside that there was something missing in my life.

It was actually my oldest son Marshall's theatrical talent that had brought us from the DC suburbs to New York City. At age eleven, he was cast in the Broadway production of *The Sound of Music*. Our move to New York opened up a whole new world to our family. Little did we know that we had a musical genius on our hands. By age thirteen, he was writing and composing music at such a high level that Stephen Schwartz, the composer of the hit musical *Wicked*, agreed to be his mentor. I often joke that it was the letter of recommendation from Schwartz that got my son into Yale.

Although my husband was a successful lawyer at a big-time New York firm, he was miserably unhappy with his work. But he was so inspired by our son's musical genius that his creativity was sparked. In the blink of an eye, he and Marshall became a father/son writing team in the highly competitive world of musical theater.

In time, and due to my son's involvement in the theater world, I became a theater producer. I supported many musicals both on and off-Broadway and produced five Broadway musicals, including *How the Grinch Stole Christmas*. I even made theatrical history by having one of my shows nominated for twelve Tony Awards and not win a single one.

Tony-nominated theater producer, thriving business owner, mother of two awesome boys, wife of a successful lawyer, founder of a theater production company…as you can imagine, those on the outside looking in thought I was living a fairy-tale life. But as we all know, looks can be deceiving.

The Widening Divide

What my friends and family did not know was that my husband and I had stopped having sex when I was thirty-two, a few years after our second son was born. As often happens with couples who lose their physical relationship, we also began to lose any intimacy in our life. Our good night cuddles started to fade away, as did kissing, with the exception of a peck on the lips. The passion we had for each other when we were first married was nonexistent.

Our king-size bed grew in dimension and there was a dividing line down the middle. We turned away from each other at night and each slept in our own prison. It didn't help matters that my husband was an insomniac and that I had restless legs. Eventually, he left our bed and started sleeping in the bottom bunk bed in my son's room.

By the time I left my marriage at age fifty, we had been sleeping in separate beds for over fifteen years. The only touch I ever received was from my children. Luckily, my youngest son, Eddie, was a cuddle-bug even into his adolescence. He also was extremely empathic and could sense my loneliness and the rift between his father and me. Eddie always knew when to give me a hug or put a hand on my arm. And he gave great shoulder massages! His gentle touch and presence kept me going through some very challenging times.

What Happened to Us?

There is a litany of reasons why my marriage fell apart, both external and internal.

On the external side, my husband felt like our move from the DC area to New York City forced him into taking a high-stakes, high-pressure legal job while he was on the cusp of receiving an MBA in Maryland. He'd hoped to leave the law and go into business, although I had my doubts it would ever happen. The move caused a tremendous amount of anger and resentment in him, which he harbored for the rest of our marriage. Ironically, it was the New York City move that ultimately helped him find and cultivate his true passion of being a writer.

Our family theater producing businesses put a tremendous amount of stress on the marriage and the family. For Marshall, the joy of writing musicals with his dad started to fade once his talent was recognized. It became clear that my husband saw Marshall as his golden ticket out of the law practice he despised more and more every day. What was once a fun sideline activity became serious; the stakes for each new musical were very high. It was excruciating to watch the power dynamics between the two of them. My teenage son, who was at the beginning of a momentous career in the arts, had to parent his father as they dealt with the inevitable disappointment that goes with the territory of creating new work.

But the worst part was the role that I played as a theater producer. It is immensely challenging to shepherd a new writer through the insular world of theater. There is a lot of disappointment along the way. No matter how brilliant, a new work that doesn't have an A level production team rarely finds its way to Broadway. Ever the bearer of bad news, I was the person who had to pass along all the constructive feedback from theater producers about why they didn't want to produce Marshall and his dad's work. The pain was beyond excruciating. What's more, it intensified the strain on my marriage, which was already veering out of control. It created a tremendous amount of tension and our conversations were fraught with anger and resentment.

We Were Doomed from the Start

In hindsight, I can now see all of the internal issues that doomed our marriage from the beginning. In choosing each other, we repeated the patterns of our childhoods. My husband replaced a strong, domineering mother, who was not affectionate and disempowered him every moment of his life, with a strong, domineering wife, who wore the pants in the family, cut him off from his sexuality, and tried to fix all of his problems. My widowed mother had taught me that love was about grief and pain. No surprise then that I chose to marry a man who was grieving over the untimely and tragic death of his older sister.

I still believe that all these issues, as insurmountable as they seemed, could have been overcome. We might still be married today, but for the fact that our sex life was completely nonexistent. Without that physical connection, what was left of our marriage was a business arrangement. We were partners in the business of raising children, partners in the theater business, but we were not partners in life.

When I think about the trajectory of the demise of my sex life, I sometimes wonder: what came first, the loss of attraction between my husband and me or my lack of interest in sex? In all fairness to my husband, I was not an easy woman to have sex with. Sex was usually painful and uncomfortable for me. I rarely, if ever, experienced sex as pleasurable. No matter how hard my husband tried to please me, I rarely got turned on. Orgasms were not in my repertoire, except a rare weak clitoral orgasm. Everything having to do with sex was a problem, including getting pregnant and suffering from such severe morning sickness that I was under a mandate of bed rest from the third trimester until I gave birth. I don't think it was humanly possible for me to feel sexually attracted to the person I associated with so much pain and discomfort.

So, we just stopped having sex.

Looking back, I understand why my body would have felt completely betrayed by anything and everything having to do with sex. Of course I shut down. Of course I was relieved to stop having sex. Yet I still felt somehow broken. And then there was the guilt about denying my husband his pleasure and feeling our relationship slip away. We rarely talked about any of this. When we did, the conversations always ended in anger and tears, which created even more distance in our relationship.

Finding a Home in Your Body

At the time, I believed my situation was an anomaly. Now I know otherwise; way too many people around the world are disconnected from their sexuality. The National Survey of Sexual Health and Behavior conducted by Indiana University in 2009 reported that 36 percent of women in their thirties did not masturbate in the last year. That number jumps to almost 50 percent for women over age fifty. The good news is that there is more awareness of the role healthy sexuality plays in our lives and more resources are available to address sexual issues.

If you're someone who finds sex challenging or feels uncomfortable with your sexuality, I've written this book for you. If you're alienated from your erotic side due to sexual abuse or trauma, you will find a healing balm in these pages. If you can't surrender to pleasure, can't sustain intimacy, or want to reclaim and feel empowered in your sexuality, consider this book a love note to you.

Before we begin your healing journey, let's look into what brought you to where you are and try to gain some understanding of why and how your challenging relationship with sex came to be.

Chapter 3

WOMEN ARE PROGRAMMED TO SAY "NO" TO SEX

The sexual revolution started over fifty years ago with the groundbreaking work of Alfred Kinsey in *The Kinsey Reports*.[1] Only in the last few decades, however, have we really had open communication about sex in the popular culture. From the affable and outrageous Dr. Ruth, who hosted the first radio show on sex in the 1980s, to the current multitude of sexperts like Emily Morse, whose *Sex with Emily* podcast has millions of fans, we both love and hate to talk about sex. Getting sex education and information from the Internet is easy, but talking about problems in our sex life is challenging. When I started my business, The Power of Pleasure, five years ago, one of my objectives was to normalize the conversation around sex. But the discomfort and shame around sex is so deep and insidious that it's even shameful to talk about our shame. No wonder clients so often comment on how valuable it was "just to have someone who I can talk to about this" after our very first session.

Sadly, most of us don't have anyone we can talk to about our sex life, our sexual problems, our sexual desires, our fetishes, and our fantasies. Talking to your partner can be highly charged and

---

1 Kinsey, Alfred C. *The Kinsey Reports*. Indiana University Press, Reprint Edition, May 22, 1988, originally published in 1948 & 1953. Print.

not without repercussions. Many couples fear that even bringing up the subject will open up a Pandora's box they will never be able to close. People often worry about bruising their partner's ego, or fear the conversation will quickly revert to blame and shame. Better not to bring it up and just put up with a bad sex life. This was certainly my experience. Every single time my ex and I tried to talk about sex, I ended up feeling guiltier, and even more broken, angry, and disconnected from him.

Some women talk to their girlfriends about their sex life or lack of one, but rarely in great detail. Most OB/GYNs and urologists are ill-equipped to provide useful advice about how to make our sex lives pain-free, better, and more pleasurable. Even couples' therapists are often extremely uncomfortable talking with clients about their sex life on any level of detail that could actually be useful. This came to me as quite a surprise initially, but in time I realized that most therapists haven't dealt with their own shame around sex.

An Oversexed, Sex-Starved Culture

The irony is that sex is talked about frankly and broadcast blatantly in popular culture. We find it everywhere…in books, movies, TV, advertising. The maxim that "Sex Sells" is true! Just take one look at a magazine advertisement for practically any lifestyle product, from sexy, sleek new cars to deodorant and lipstick. Sex entices us and is also the forbidden fruit driving our desires and wallets.

You would think we'd be sexually open in a society that constantly throws sex in our face. In fact, the opposite is true. The United States is a sex-negative and sex-starved nation. The latest statistics about the lack of sex in this country are horrifying.

According to "The National Survey of Sexual Health and Behavior" (2010), the average married couple has sex about once a week. Twenty percent of couples are only having sex once a month, which is considered a sexless marriage. I suspect those numbers are significantly underreported. This study does not account for the large number of men and women who stay in their marriage for financial reasons and/or "for the children," but have completely unsatisfying sex lives. Sex workers report that the vast majority of men who see them for sensual massage or escort services are happily married men living in virtually sexless marriages.

Sexless Marriage vs. Upsetting the Apple Cart

I asked myself many times why I chose to stay in my marriage. In my thirties, when I still had a libido, I toyed with having an affair with a work colleague, but we both chickened out. That should have been a clear signal that my marriage was in trouble, but I ignored it. We had small kids, a good family life, and we were constantly trading up to nicer cars and homes. Why upset the apple cart? Even when my kids were older, and we weren't having sex or sleeping in the same room, I had a hard time calling it quits. At one point, I created a five-year plan to leave my marriage that I shared with one of my best friends, who was also contemplating divorce.

Sexless marriages are so pervasive in our society that there seems to be an attempt in some sectors to "normalize" the fact that couples stop having sex, especially when they get into their fifties and beyond. Recently the *Huffington Post*, which is arguably the most sex-positive mainstream media outlet in the US, published an article titled, "Over 50 and in a Sexless Marriage: Don't Despair."

Essentially, the author's position was that people could thrive in a sexless marriage. But there was something missing in the article that I feel is important to take into account. It's true: couples often decide not to engage in sex. However, the majority of the time, the decision is forced on one of the partners. In fact, a common scenario is that one partner loses interest, becomes unresponsive, and starts to avoid anything to do with sex. The still-desirous party keeps trying for a while, then gets tired of rejection and simply gives up. Often this unfolds with no discussion at all, much less a conscious decision.

Where Did My Libido Go?

Unfortunately, for 90 percent of the clients that I've worked with, it is the woman who loses her desire to have sex. While each situation is unique, there are some common causes:

- Women are socialized to say "no" to sex
- We hold shame and fear around fully sexually expressing ourselves
- Motherhood transforms us from sexual beings to maternal beings
- Sex becomes boring and rote
- We are not sufficiently aroused and don't experience enough pleasure
- Women are often not connected to their sexuality

In these and many other ways, we women are essentially programmed to say "no" to sex. In contrast, men literally wear their sexual arousal equipment on the outside of their body. As teenage boys, they were constantly getting aroused and getting erections, often at inconvenient times, but it made their sexuality front and center. Men also receive many more positive messages around sex. "Always use protection" and "don't get her pregnant," while you "go out and sow your wild oats." High-fives in the locker room after "scoring" the night before are part and parcel of male culture. Teenage boys grow up with porn, which turns women into sex objects and creates unrealistic expectations about body parts and what sex really is like.

Given this socialization, there is no surprise that when I ask men how often they think about wanting to have sex, the most common answer is, "Multiple times a day." Women, on the other hand, typically say that they think about sex at most once or twice a month! Why are we so disconnected from our desire?

"Keep Your Legs Shut!"

First of all, Mother Nature designed our sexual parts to be less visible and accessible. While we have a vast and complex arousal network, it is almost entirely on the inside of our body, with the exception of our nipples. Even a woman's clitoris is 75 percent internal—the only parts that are exposed (the head and shaft) are covered by a hood. Women need lots of warm-up and touch to get aroused, whereas a man is likely to become easily aroused if he has any physical stimulation on his cock.

We were taught that sex is tied to our menstrual cycle, a subject that for many young girls is painful, shameful and embarrassing. I know I am not alone in having experienced embarrassing "accidents." Many of the women I have worked with have shameful memories about their periods. The situation is compounded by the fact that many of us did not have mothers who were particularly helpful or empathetic. Being handed a pad and told to read some instructions reinforces the belief that sex and our periods are dirty. This creates further distance between our bodies and our sexuality.

For the most part, sex education for women focuses on preventing pregnancy, protection against STIs, and—for many in this country—abstinence. We are told to "keep our legs shut" because the only thing boys want is to get into our pants. Sexually active teenage girls are called "easy" and are slut-shamed by both their female and male peers. Pleasure is not mentioned anywhere in the sex education curriculum.

For women, fear and shame around sexual expression is rampant. We have a belief that expressing our pleasure by making loud noises is not appropriate or ladylike and threatens our idealized view of how women are supposed to behave. Sexually expressed women are depicted as vixens, sirens, or femmes fatales. Every girl watching *Sex and the City* wants to grow up to be "Carrie," not "Samantha." Historically, sexually expressed women have been burned at the stake or tarred and feathered. And we continue to be slut-shamed in public and in private. When is the last time you heard of a sexually expressive woman being elevated in the media in a positive way and not sensationalized? This sexual atmosphere carries over into the bedroom. It prevents us from being able to fully surrender and connect to our desires and our pleasure, making it impossible for us to lead an orgasmic life.

Good Girl Madonna, Bad Girl Whore

The Madonna/Whore complex is yet another influence that causes women to be disconnected from their sexuality. It also tends to cause sexual problems in long-term relationships. In the psychoanalytic literature, Sigmund Freud argues that the Madonna/Whore complex is caused by a split between the affectionate and the sexual aspects of male desire. Men tend to categorize women as either good girl Madonnas who are pure, innocent, and virginal, or bad girl Whores who are sexually expressive, indiscriminate, and aggressive. Men want to marry and have kids with the Madonna, but are sexually attracted to the Whore.

While much has been written about the Madonna/Whore complex and its impact on men, it also has an enormous effect on women. "Should I have sex with him on the first date?" is a common question single women ask themselves, a question that is made ever more difficult to answer when there is lots of chemistry. We fear that if we do have sex, we will get labeled as the Whore and won't be considered long-term relationship material. He will disregard our intense passion and chemistry the minute he encounters the nice girl who meets his ideal image of a wife.

The Madonna/Whore complex often influences our choice of long-term partner and how we behave sexually once we are married. Before the wedding, sex is lustful, playful, experimental, and highly erotic. Not long after the wedding, it's all boring, vanilla sex. I often talk with women who in their single days were fully erotically expressive and enjoyed their sexuality with the "bad boy" types, but ended up marrying a "good boy." Then, out of fear that their true sexual nature will cause their more conservative partner to leave, they repress their sexuality and succumb to boring sex. No one is happy about that. Ironically, it's usually the "good boys" who lust for playful, hot sex and often end up seeking it outside of marriage.

The Madonna/Whore complex also shows up as women move into motherhood and often end up disconnecting from their sexuality. Motherhood consumes us, especially in the early years. Our identity as a sexual woman and a lover gets subsumed under our new identity as a mom. New mothers often complain that they used to love it when their husband sucked and fondled their breasts, but it became a turn-off once they had nursed a child. All of a sudden our breasts transform from sex organs into milk machines, and it's often hard to lose that association.

Good Sex Begets More Good Sex

If you are like most women, you are not experiencing nearly enough pleasure during lovemaking. As a result, sex stops being a priority. Given our tremendous orgasmic capacity and pleasure potential, this is a tragedy. Our ability to experience long, powerful multiple orgasms that bring us to another level of consciousness far exceeds what most men can experience. What few women and even fewer men understand is that a woman's desire for sex follows her arousal, which is completely the opposite of a man, whose arousal follows his desire. The more we women have sex, the more we want sex. But in order to be interested in sex in the first place, women must become aroused enough for our desire to kick in. We will get into this in more depth in Chapter 13.

When a woman starts to experience physical pleasure on a regular basis, her desire for sex will go through the roof. But most women never even come close to experiencing sex as pleasurable. In fact, women often have intercourse long before they are sufficiently aroused. In the best-case scenario, this makes for sex that is "only OK" and, in the worst-case scenario, outright painful.

I totally get it. If sex is "only OK," and you are doing it more to please your partner or out of obligation than to please yourself, it falls low on your ever-growing to-do list. If it starts to feel like work rather than play, resentment builds up. If you are putting up with touch that really doesn't feel good—which is the number one complaint that women have about their sex life—you start harboring even more anger, disappointment, and regret that further disconnects you from your partner and your sex life. If you, like most women, desire strong masculine energy and sometimes want to be "taken," with consent, and your partner comes to you with sweet, "good boy" energy that does not turn you on, you start losing attraction to him. All of this creates a downward spiral, further tamps down your desire, and disconnects you from your sexuality. But the number one reason that holds us back from experiencing pleasure and connecting to our desire and the true potential of living an orgasmic life is SHAME. In the next chapter, we will explore all of the ways in which shame shuts us down and why it happens in the first place.

Chapter 4

SHAME: THE NASTIEST FIVE-LETTER WORD IN THE UNIVERSE

Most of us don't spend a lot of time thinking about shame. We know the feeling of embarrassment when we say or do something stupid, but shame is more elusive, not really on our radar screen. There's a reason for this: shame is so deeply repressed we can't even access it.

Therein lies the problem: shame is something we don't talk about. It's so insidious that we can't even see it for what it is and rarely bring it up except in a special context such as therapy. And yet shame drives much of our behavior, especially with regard to our sexuality. Its influence is both powerful and harmful, which is why I consider it the nastiest five-letter word in our universe.

The Shame/Pleasure Paradox

If shame is what holds us back from enjoying sex and experiencing pleasure, where exactly does it come from? After all, human beings are designed to experience pleasure. Think about babies. For a short period of time, they do live an orgasmic life. Babies and toddlers freely explore and touch their bodies with wonderment and joy. They love to put their toes in their mouth, coo when they are breastfeeding or drinking from a bottle, touch themselves all over, and freely express pleasure. As we get older, our spontaneous expression of joy lessens as we are compelled by our environment to rein in our pleasure-seeking impulses, especially those that are sexual in nature. Little ones naturally reach for their genitals and are often subtly or overtly reprimanded for doing so.

It's an odd paradox, given that we have over ten thousand nerve endings in our genitals. It would seem as though our bodies are designed to experience sexual pleasure. Did you know that, inch for inch, your clitoris has as many nerve endings as a man's penis? Unlike the penis, the clitoris does not serve a specific role in reproduction. The only purpose of the clitoris is for us to experience pleasure. Of course, experiencing pleasure encourages procreation, but a clitoral orgasm does not get you pregnant! Pleasure and orgasm have many health benefits: reducing stress, improving sleep, pain relief, boosting your immune system, and providing a natural antidepressant.

Our bodies are a source of pleasure, and our physiology supports the argument that we are meant to experience pleasure. But when we get older and want to touch ourselves, an element of shame often seeps in, spoiling our experience of bodily pleasure. This paradox creates tension around our sexuality. As you will see, sexual shame comes from a variety of different sources.

Ancient Cultures Were Sex-Positive

If we look at sexuality from a historical perspective, we find that attitudes toward sex in many ancient cultures were actually quite positive. According to Paul Chrystal, author of *In Bed with the Ancient Greeks: Sex & Sexuality in Ancient Greece*:

> ...love and sex were inextricably connected with the creation of the Earth, the heavens, and the underworld. Greek myth

was a theogony of incest, murder, polygamy, and intermarriage in which eroticism and fertility were elemental; they were there right from the start, demonstrating woman's essential reproductive role in securing the cosmos, extending the human race, and ensuring the fecundity of nature." Many ancient religions also worshipped sex. In ancient Hindu temples all over the world, we find statues of Lingams (penises) and Yonis (vulvas) worshipping the God Shiva and Goddess Parvati.[2]

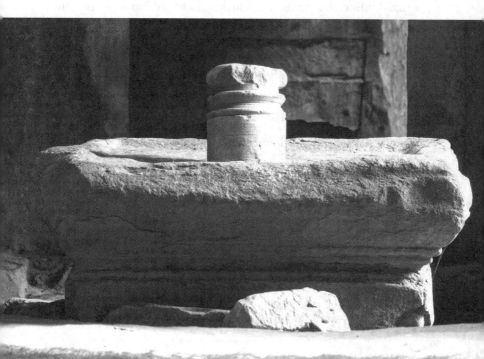

Yoni Lingam Statute, Siem Riep, Cambodia, Angkor Wat
Temple Ruins, 12th Century

2 Paul Chrystal, *In Bed with the Ancient Greeks: Sex & Sexuality in Ancient Greece*. Amberly Publishing, 2016. Print.

It was the Judeo-Christian religion that vilified sex. Adam and Eve were shamed for their nakedness, accused of "original sin" for eating the "forbidden apple" and banished from the Garden of Eden, that paradise wherein pleasure and joy were one's birthright. We have been paying the price of their banishment and carrying the weight of their shame ever since.

Shame and Your Sexual Blueprint

To understand where our shame comes from, we have to examine our sexual blueprint. Similar to an architectural blueprint that shows all the details of the plumbing, electricity, drywall, windows, and doors that make up a building, you have a sexual blueprint comprised of all the early life experiences that make up your sense of yourself as a sexual being. I call it a blueprint to emphasize the impact of the early experiences that govern your relationship with your own sexuality as well as how you relate to members of the opposite or the same sex. The elements of your sexual blueprint include:

- Messages you received about sex as a child from parents, other adults, and society
- Early childhood sexual exploration with yourself and/ or others
- Your first sexual experiences
- Relationships with your mother and father or primary caregiver
- Seminal events that impacted your body image
- Religious ideology or indoctrination

How these messages impact you differs for everyone, but we all experience shame…that is a part of human existence. Let me give you an example of how this plays out. When I was growing up, I had a dog whose name was Lucky. He was a yappy, high-strung, neurotic Yorkshire terrier; we did not have the best relationship. Lucky often barked at and nipped me. He loved to hide under my bed and then growl at me when I tried to get him to come out. When I was nine years old, Lucky started to lick my private parts while I was lying in bed at night. I experienced a lot of pleasure from the sensation of the dog's tongue on my pussy. I also knew from earlier experiences that I would be punished if my mother caught me. So the pleasure I experienced was colored with fear, anxiety, and shame.

Fast-forward eighteen years. Is there any wonder that I was really uncomfortable with oral sex and could never relax enough to experience it as pleasurable? Not until I slowly brought this memory to consciousness in my forties and shared it with a group of people in a workshop was I finally able to heal my shame and begin enjoying oral sex. Interestingly, when I shared my shame story through tears and shaking during that workshop, another woman shared that she'd been sexually aroused as a child by rubbing against her cat! What a relief! For decades, I thought there was something wrong with me; that I was broken, sexually deranged, or maybe even into bestiality.

The most important lesson I learned from the workshop is that the only way to normalize the conversation about sex is to normalize the conversation about shame. There are many ways to do that, but writing about it, talking about it, and sharing our experience with others are powerful first steps toward healing shame. Later on in this chapter you will get to explore your own sexual blueprint, but for now let's look at some other real-life examples of how our sexual shame impacts our sexuality.

Body Shame: Jessica's Story

Jessica came to see me because she was uncomfortable touching herself and was not able to have an orgasm. She grew up in a fairly open and sex-positive environment within her family. Jessica was a tomboy and loved playing with the neighborhood boys. For years, on warm summer days, she ran around topless, just like her friends did. She loved the freedom of being bare-chested and feeling the air on her skin. Her parents were totally fine with this, and Jessica continued to experience her freedom. But when Jessica turned ten, with budding breasts, things changed.

It was a beautiful, warm summer day, and like always, Jessica ran outside the house without a shirt on to play basketball with the boys. Her mother, who had been running errands, pulled onto the street, took one look at Jessica and her budding breasts, stopped the car, and demanded that she go inside the house and "put a shirt on right this second." Jessica's body shame was exacerbated in middle school when a teacher told her that she needed to "sit like a lady" and keep her legs closed.

In middle school Jessica gained a lot of weight, probably to hide herself from her own body. The disconnection from her body increased when she was later shamed for being "fat" by her aunts and uncles. It was carried over to her adult life as an inability to enjoy touching and appreciating her own body. Over time, Jessica was able to accept that the shame and negative image she had about her body were from her childhood, had no basis in fact, and no longer served her. As she began connecting with her own feminine self, she became more loving and compassionate to herself and her body. Eventually she was able to enjoy touching and pleasuring herself and experienced her first orgasm.

Delayed Ejaculation Shame: Jeff's Story

Jeff came to see me after a nasty divorce. He was afraid of being intimate with women and was particularly concerned about delayed ejaculation, meaning he could get fully aroused but not come. When I asked Jeff about his first sexual experience, he told me this story.

> I was seventeen when I lost my virginity. I was one of the last of my group of friends and felt a lot of peer pressure to get laid. There was this girl, Jackie, who had a lot of experience and came on to me at a party. I wasn't attracted to her, but she put her hand on my cock when we were dancing, and I felt excited. She took me into a back bedroom and we fucked. It went on for about a half an hour, and while it felt really good, I couldn't come. Jackie made fun of me and even told her girlfriends about it. I felt like all her friends looked at me in a different way after that. Like I was not a real man.

And thus, shame became a cornerstone of Jeff's sexual blueprint. Jeff repeated this pattern when he started dating after the divorce. He'd agree to have sex with a woman when he really wasn't that turned on and didn't feel connected. Then, when he couldn't ejaculate, he'd think himself inadequate and feel deeply ashamed. Once Jeff learned to relax during sex and developed stronger boundaries so he could say "no" to women he was not attracted to, he was able to enjoy making love, and his problem with delayed ejaculation went away.

My own sexual shame runs fairly deep in my blueprint and was etched into my sense of myself at a fairly early age. As a young child, I was pretty sexual and often played doctor with my friends. One day I was over at my best friend Josephine's house. We were two bubbly first-graders pretending we were doctors and exploring each other's vaginas. This was one of our favorite games. When Josephine's mother walked into the room, her face turned bright red. She scolded us, immediately called my mother to tell her what had happened, and demanded she come pick me up right away. My mother, who never showed any connection to her own sexuality, couldn't even talk to me except to say it was a "bad thing" that I could never do again. After that incident, Josephine's mother would not let us have play dates anymore. At the end of first grade, Josephine and her family moved away. I was heartbroken to lose my friend and believed it was my fault she had to move away. Thus began the association between my vagina and painful disappointment.

EXERCISE: SEXUAL BLUEPRINT

Think about your own childhood and what kind of messages you received about sex from your parents, other adults and society. Reflect on the following questions. Write down any images that come to mind. Writing down what you notice gives your memory permission to open up and deliver more information about a particular incident or scene.

- Did you see your parents hold hands and touch each other? How often?
- Did your parents kiss in front of you? Were their kisses tender or perfunctory?
- Were you allowed to crawl into your parents' bed to cuddle?
- Did you ever see your parents or other adults naked? What were the circumstances?
- Did your parents make you hide your eyes if there was a romantic scene on TV?
- When did you first learn about sex?
- Was there ever any discussion about sex in your family?
- What impact do you think these messages have had on your own sexuality?
- At what age do you remember first exploring your body and genitals and experiencing some sensation? Did you do this alone or with a sibling or friend?
- Were you ever afraid that you might get caught exploring or touching yourself? If you did have the experience of being caught, describe what happened and how it made you feel.

How does your sexual blueprint impact your adult sexual relationships? Did you notice that so many of the beliefs that you have about sex come from others? If you were to rid yourself of those false beliefs, how would that impact your sexuality? Your sexual blueprint is key to understanding and changing your relationship with sex and intimacy.

My father's death when I was three greatly impacted my sexual blueprint. Not only did my mother never remarry, she never dated and never invited a man, other than a relative, over to our house. Sex was never discussed. My mother so hated touch that she wouldn't get a manicure and took no pleasure in keeping her own nails perfectly shaped. She could barely talk to me when I got my period at the age of eleven, other than to reinforce the overriding message: "sex is bad and dirty." My only knowledge of romantic love was from what I saw in the movies and read in books, which caused me to idolize men.

Shame from Inappropriate Attraction: Tim's Story

Growing up in a sexually open household also has its challenges. Tim, age forty-three, was unable to sustain healthy relationships with women because he was obsessed with his mother and constantly fantasized about her. He grew up in a household where nudity was acceptable. His mother had always walked around the house naked and this never presented a problem, until he entered puberty. Tim had his first erotic experience when he got a hard-on while looking at his mother with her breasts exposed. His mother noticed Tim's erection and said, "I'm flattered by all your attention." Tim also saw that his mother's nipples had become erect and he realized that she was also turned on. This reinforced his sexual attraction to her.

His mother squandered a perfect opportunity to remove the shame from the situation by simply telling Tim that it's normal for a boy to get an erection when he sees a naked woman's body. She also should have realized that her days of walking around naked in front of Tim were over. Instead his attention played into her own sexual desires, creating an inappropriate mother-son dynamic.

Religious and cultural beliefs can also have a huge impact on our sexuality, particularly in Christianity and Islam. I work with a lot of men and women from India, Asia, and the Middle East. Many of them grew up in very sex-negative cultures where women are supposed to be virgins when they marry. Women are looked down upon if they dress in a feminine or sexy way. Girls receive a lot of negative messages and are often shamed for expressing their sexuality.

Sexually Repressed Shame: Anya's Story

Anya's family is from Iran. Sex was not talked about in her home and her mother put the kibosh on even the slightest hint of sexual expression. One day she and her mother were driving in a car and she saw a woman on the back of a motorcycle being driven by a man. The woman's hair was flying and she was holding on to him very tightly. Feeling excited by this vision she said out loud, "Oh, I wish that was me." Out of nowhere, she felt a slap across her face. "She's a slut," said her mother with disgust. "And you will be too if you do that!"

Anya told me this story during a session. I'd been giving her some featherlight touch on her arms and she started to feel a little pleasure in her body, which I could sense from her breathing. But the minute she felt that pleasure, she froze up and started crying. When I asked her what was going on she told me that she heard her mother's voice in her head telling her that she was a slut and that pleasure was shameful. Pleasure and shame had collapsed into a single experience for her. This prevented her from ever being able to touch herself or experience an orgasm. Once she realized why she was blocked, she was able to accept pleasure and eventually have orgasms.

On the opposite end of the spectrum from shame caused by sexual repression is the projection of shame onto women who are sexually expressive, what we call "slut-shaming." Women who are sexually open, available, and have lots of sex are stigmatized as "loose" and too free with their bodies. One of the insidious messages young women receive is, "You don't want to open your legs for too many men!" Sadly, slut-shaming most often occurs woman-to-woman.

Shame Around Experiencing Desire: Bob's Story

Another example of shame around desire showed up with Bob. He was ashamed about how highly sexually excitable he was, walking around with a hard-on much of the day. Even the calming breathing exercises I taught him turned him on. From age eight to age twelve, Bob had ongoing sexual experiences with his older sister wherein he would touch or suck her breasts but never received touch in return. While this was a big turn-on for Bob and left him with an erection, he was also confused. He felt both excited and anxious about being caught. Shame seeped in because he knew what he was doing was wrong, but he also felt helpless against his sister's advances. Bob also had a volatile relationship with his rageaholic father. He got aroused and had a hard-on whenever his father exploded at him. Over time, he began to associate erections and arousal with emotions of fear, anxiety, excitement, sadness, and anger. Layered over all of this was shame. Through our sessions, Bob began to understand that he used his arousal to distract himself from his emotions. Once Bob learned to express his emotions, his sexual arousal became more appropriate to the situation.

Masturbation and Shame

As children, many of us got caught masturbating by a parent or another adult figure. They typically let their disapproval be known and we were reprimanded: teasing, scolding, looks of disdain, even mild to severe punishments. This was certainly my experience with my friend Josephine in first grade. I never felt the same about Josephine after that incident. The feelings from being caught and the disapproval made me feel embarrassed, guilty, confused and very upset. This common experience leads to shame and the inability to freely express our sexuality and to experience pleasure.

Masturbation Shame and Disassociation from Pleasure: Delia's Story

Delia was experiencing orgasm challenges. While her body went through the normal physiological response to arousal and orgasm, (heavier breathing, increased heart rate, flushed face) she did not experience much sensation in her body when she was aroused. One day, I was giving Delia a bodywork session intended to help her open up to receiving sensual touch and I noticed that the fingers on her right hand were moving in a pattern that mimicked masturbation. When I brought this to her attention, she recalled the shame she felt when, as a young girl, her mother barged into her room, smelled her fingers, and punished her for touching herself. The pleasure of masturbation turned into shame, and while Delia continued to masturbate as a child, she never again experienced pleasure. This continued into adulthood, and Delia started to disassociate from any pleasurable sensations during sex. Even though her body responded to sensual touch, she did not feel aroused and felt numb around her pussy.

As Delia began to deal with her shame, she became much more aware and present to sensations and her arousal and ultimately was able to fully experience orgasm.

Masturbation Shame and Early Ejaculation: Keith's Story

In men, problems with early ejaculation are often associated with getting caught masturbating in adolescence. Keith was an only child with a very controlling mother, who was constantly checking up on him. The bathroom, the only room in the house with a lock on the door, was Keith's refuge from his mother, and the only safe place for him to masturbate. Eventually his mother caught on to this. She began monitoring his time in the bathroom, constantly knocking on the door and asking him if everything was all right. Fearful of her interference, Keith learned how to come very quickly, usually within two minutes of stimulation. This became his normal response and plagued him into adulthood and marriage.

In my work with men and women, I am always surprised by the impact of negative responses to a child's natural curiosity and tendency to touch themselves "down there." The mere act of swatting a little boy's hand away from his crotch quickly sends the message that touching yourself is wrong. These messages stick with us and are often further reinforced by societal and religious messages about masturbation.

Body Shame: A Generalized, Cultural Disorder

Body shame is an experience common to almost all women and many men surrounding our looks, our weight, the size of our breasts, cocks, thighs, butts, pussies…the list can go on forever. The constant barrage of unrealistic media images of perfect bodies and body parts continues to play a huge role in our own body image issues. I have worked with so many men who have shame because their penises don't measure up to the ones they see in pornography, many of which have been digitally enhanced.

For women, body shame is the number one reason that we are held back from enjoying sex and creates disconnection from our desires. Women tend to "spectate" during sex, i.e., we are constantly thinking about and imagining what our bodies look like while we are having sex. This takes us out of the experience and into our heads. I know I've done this, and I'm sure you have as well. I've gone so far as to require that the mirror in my room be covered during sex because I was unhappy with the way my body looked.

Body shame prevents you from fully expressing yourself sexually. Maybe you have sex under the covers or with the lights out so that your partner doesn't see your body. Body shame creates unhealthy habits, such as constant dieting and eating disorders. You might even sabotage every first date just to avoid exposing your body to someone else.

Body shame often makes us feel like we're not loveable, not sexy, and not worthy of someone's attention. It also causes many unnecessary surgeries such as penile implants, breast enhancements and reductions, and labiaplasty, a common form of plastic surgery for women.

Many of us first experience body shame in our early adolescence, just as our bodies are changing. Hormones do funny things to bodies, but there is little compassion for this, and cruel comments from others can cut right through us. When Joelle went to sleep-away camp at age fourteen, she gained fifteen pounds over the summer. Excited about returning home to see her boyfriend, she has a vivid memory of how shocked he was when he met her at the door. She will never forget the look on his face. Rather than inviting her into the house to talk with his parents as he normally did, he quickly ushered her upstairs, sending shame and negative messages to her about her body. To cope with the body shame, Joelle resorted to massive fasts and dieting and ended up with an eating disorder in college.

Postpartum women are particularly burdened by body shame, and it is part of the reason so many of us lose interest in sex after giving birth. Unfortunately, I have seen some women whose partners exacerbate their shame by continuing to buy them clothes that are one or two sizes too small as an "incentive" to get back to pre-baby weight. I personally consider that yet another form of shaming.

Exercise: Body Talk

We all have issues around our body image, parts of our bodies that we don't like and wish were different.

1. List seven of your favorite body parts.

2. If you could change one body part, what would it be and how would you change it? List all the ways that changing that one body part would change your life.

3. Look at your list from question two. For each statement, ask yourself, *Is this really true?* If the answer is *yes*, reflect on what other changes you could make in your life to have the same desired outcome.

4. Take time for reflection. Close your eyes and take a few deep breaths. Recall a time when someone said something about your body that made you feel ashamed, inadequate, or hurt your feelings. Take a few minutes to really go back into your memory and notice what types of sensation you might be feeling in your body. Describe the sensations you had in your body when you felt this shame.

5. Ask a trusted partner, friend, or family member if you can share this story with them because you are working on getting rid of your body shame. After you have shared the story, go back into your memory and notice whether anything has changed in your experience of it.

Too Big, Too Small: Sex Organ Shame

In my case, while growing up, I had huge issues about the size of my breasts, which just seemed way out of proportion to the rest of my body. My mother never thought to make sure I was wearing a bra with decent support, so they bounced all over the place. I wasn't upset about this because I assumed it was normal, until I found out it wasn't. It was a warm spring morning, so I was wearing only a tight T-shirt as I walked along the busy street on my way to school. A red pick-up truck drew up beside me. Workmen in the back of the truck pointed to me and called out "Hey, big tits," while giving me very sexual looks. I was devastated. My face turned bright red; I started crying and ran away. For several months afterward, I made my mother drive me to school. Every time I passed that corner, I felt sick to my stomach. It took years for me to overcome this body image issue and realize that my breasts are one of my most valuable assets.

Many men also suffer from body shame. *The Guardian* published an article, "Me and My Penis: 100 Men Reveal All,"[3] an interview with Laura Dodsworth, author of *Manhood: The Bare Reality* (Pinter & Martin, LTD, 2017), a new book about men and sexuality. The author photographed one hundred men's penises and then talked to them about body image issues and sexuality. What surprised her most? "A lot more men feel a sense of shame or anxiety about their size, or an aspect of their performance, than I would have thought. What really moved me is how much that shame and inadequacy had bled into different parts of their life."

---

3   Laura Dodsworth, "Me and My Penis: 100 Men Reveal All." *The Guardian*. May 27, 2017. Accessed June 01, 2018. https://www.theguardian.com/lifeandstyle/2017/may/27/me-and-my-penis-100-men-reveal-all.

Internet pornography causes lots of cock shame. You have no idea how many men feel inadequate because they compare their completely normal size penis to the lengths and girths of porn stars. Men, the cocks in pornography are not normal! They are either digitally enhanced or are injected with drugs to induce an erection and increase engorgement. A 2015 study in the British Journal of Urological Surgeons reported that an average size erect penis is 5.1 inches in length and 4.6 inches in girth (circumference). A 6.5-inch penis is in the ninety-fifth percentile; most porn stars are in the ninety-ninth percentile of penis size! And the truth is that most women don't really care about the size of a man's cock, as long as he knows how to use it. In fact, a man with a smaller cock can have quite the advantage when it comes to giving a woman an internal G-spot orgasm with his penis if he learns how.

Cock shame comes up for boys in many different circumstances as they are growing up. The proverbial locker room cock size comparison has done quite a number on many men. But the majority of cock shaming comes from women who complain about the size of their partner's cock, or even worse, compare one cock to another.

Cock Size Shame: Jim's Story

Jim was only twenty-nine years old, but was having erection problems. He was referred to me because he was considering having a penile implant, which should be unnecessary in a healthy twenty-nine-year-old man. What was really going on for Jim? In Jim's last relationship, his girlfriend had complained about the size of his cock, saying he was smaller than other men she had been with. Jim started a regimen of useless supplements (they do not make the cock bigger), as well as a series of intense exercises to stretch his cock. He completely bought into the notion that his cock size was inadequate. This shame had a huge impact on him.

When I first met him, he had low energy, his shoulders were bent over, and you could tell that he was carrying a big weight. He was struggling with school and his career. In one of our early sessions, we measured the size of his erect penis, and I showed him this chart indicating average penis size.

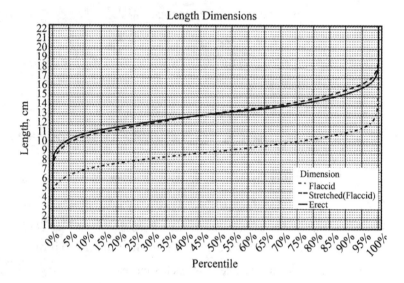

Distribution of Penis Size from a sample of 15,000 Men
Average erect penis is 5.16 inches (13.12 cm)

I could literally see the weight lift from his shoulders as it dawned on him that his six-inch erect penis was way above average. By the end of the session he was standing tall and beginning to feel his own power. I also gave Jim lots of compliments about his cock.

Ladies: Men Need to Hear Compliments about Their Cock

Try some of these on:

- You have a beautiful cock
- I am so honored to touch your cock
- I love the way your cock tastes and smells
- I love your cock and the way it feels against my skin, in my mouth, in my pussy
- Thank you for sharing your cock with me

You have no idea how emotional men can get when they hear these compliments coming from you. Jim recently contacted me to thank me for the relaxation skills I taught him, which have been helpful in his new career in the adult film entertainment industry. He is definitely over his cock shame!

Pussy Shame

Women are certainly not immune from genital shame. Many women hate the look and smell of their vaginas. More so than men, many women have a really difficult time touching themselves, and a huge percentage have never looked at their own vaginas.

My Vagina is Normal!: Annie's Story

It was a beautiful October day and I was enjoying a break between clients when my phone rang. A woman on the other end started crying the minute she heard my voice. It took a moment for me to realize that this was not a prank call but someone in real distress. Annie told me that she was scheduled to have labia plastic surgery in a week. She was having second thoughts and had read one of my blog posts begging women not to have the surgery. "I hate the way I look down there," she said. "My lips hang down, I have all this flesh covering me. I don't feel sexy and it turns off my partner." In between sobs, she told me that she never touched her pussy with her hands and rubbed against a sheet to masturbate. "I don't look like any of the women in the porn we watch!" she cried.

When Annie came to see me, I shared with her the book *Femalia* by Joani Blank, which contains pictures of hundreds of vaginas, in all different shapes, colors, and sizes. She was shocked to see the variety of vaginas and even identified a few that were shaped like hers.[4] We also read about "female genital anatomy types" from *The Sexual Practices of Quodoushka: Teachings from the Nagual Tradition.* Quodoushka is a Native American based sacred sexuality practice, much like Tantra. They have identified nine different female and male genital types, all of which are given animal names and powers (e.g., Wolf Woman, Deer Woman). According to the tradition, each type has its own set of characteristics: physical, emotional, temperament, sexual preferences, and orgasmic qualities.[5] A big smile broke out on Annie's face when she read the description of the Antelope Woman. "That's me!" she exclaimed, relieved that her pussy was normal.

One of the most powerful exercises I do with women is having them look at their vaginas in a mirror and begin to explore the

---

4   Joani Blank, *Femalia*. Down There Press, 1993. Print.

5   Amara Charles, *The Sexual Practices of Quodoushka: Teachings from the Nagual Tradition*. Destiny Books, 2011. Print.

wonders of the "yoniverse." Yoni is a Sanskrit word for vagina and means a lotus flower. I lovingly call a woman's whole vulva, of which the vagina is really only the internal canal, her "yoniverse." Layla Martin, a modern-day Tantra guru, recently did a wonderful video where they took pictures of women's Yonis. They compared a woman's reaction to seeing a photo of her own Yoni with her partner's reaction to seeing the same photo. It was striking how critical women were of their Yonis compared to their partners. If you are considering having vaginoplasty or labiaplasty, please reconsider. They are painful procedures that create scar tissue and eliminate thousands of nerve endings, significantly reducing your sensation and orgasmic potential.

Sexual Fetishism

I really don't like the word fetish because it labels sexual preferences as normal and not normal. I believe that anything that gives you pleasure and is done with a fully consenting adult partner is normal. If a golden shower, cross dressing, flogging, or licking someone's foot turns you on, more power to you. Kinky sex is still sex and gives many people, myself included, a tremendous amount of pleasure. But what if you feel tremendous shame about a sexual desire that you believe is outside the norm?

Cross Dressing and Submissive Shame: Ralph's Story

Ralph, a thirty-five-year-old CFO of a successful company, and his wife came to see me for help to get their sex life back on track. When Ralph filled out my new client form, he said he had a secret he did not want to share with his wife. In an individual session, Ralph told me that he loves to wear lingerie and has a rich fantasy life around being submissive. I assured Ralph that his fantasies were perfectly normal and not at all uncommon, but Ralph had a tremendous amount of shame around his desires. His wife knew about his interest in wearing women's underwear and seemed comfortable with that, but she did not know about his submissive desires.

In order to overcome his shame, Ralph had to look deeply at the beliefs his Catholic upbringing had instilled in him, as well as his difficulty connecting with his emotions and a tendency to numb out with alcohol or marijuana. He also worked at an extraordinarily stressful job and had a complicated relationship with his father, who headed up the family company. I completely understood why Ralph was so turned on by being a submissive, which is commonplace for powerful men. It was the one place where he could totally surrender and not be required to make a single decision. Ralph's wife was totally willing to embrace his fantasy of being submissive, but he had a hard time letting go of his judgment of himself. Over the course of a year, Ralph and I met regularly so that he could explore his desires in a safe, nonjudgmental setting. Self-love and acceptance came gradually, and he was eventually able to share his fantasy with his wife, who accepted it—and him—completely.

Accepting your own shame is one of the prerequisites for living an orgasmic life. While you may not be able to rid yourself completely of all your shame, understanding where it comes from and its impact on your sexuality is a major step toward embracing it. Your shame is just another part of you that needs to be loved.

Chapter 5

SEXUAL ABUSE AND TRAUMA

Survivors of sexual abuse, especially childhood sexual abuse, will almost always struggle with their sexuality and intimate relationships. Sexual abuse strips away our ability to trust other people, as well as ourselves. Many victims blame themselves for their abuser's behavior. Abuse survivors often do not feel safe in their bodies, and any type of sexual touch can easily trigger a traumatic reaction.

Sexual abuse is so rampant in our country, you would think there would be a national outcry—we'd certainly see one if the problem was in any area other than sex. In the United States, one in four women have experienced abuse such as nonconsensual touch, according to the National Sexual Violence Resource Center. Those numbers are staggering and incomprehensible, but most women who come to see me for healing work have experienced some form of abuse. While most abusers of girls and women are men, many girls and women are abused by mothers, aunts, or babysitters. For the purpose of this chapter, I am going to focus on the more common scenario: a male sexually abusing a female.

Overt and Covert Abuse

Sexual abuse comes in all different forms. Overt abuse involving nonconsensual physical touch is most common. Many women also experience covert abuse, however; for example:

- Visual or verbal abuse by male family members or trusted authority figures
- Inappropriate comments
- "Peeping Tom" incidents
- Indecent exposure
- An adult male intentionally looking at a naked woman or girl in an inappropriate way

This type of covert abuse is often disguised to appear seemingly innocent or accidental. An example is what happened to Jane when she was a young girl. Every time she took a shower, her stepfather would conveniently "forget" something in the bathroom. Maria's father would find excuses to look under the table for something when she was wearing a short skirt or nightgown. Just like nonconsensual physical touch, this type of activity causes women to feel dirty, unsafe, and even ashamed in the presence of men.

Women who have experienced overt sexual abuse have a wounding so deep that it leaves indelible marks on their physical and emotional bodies and psyches, often causing a traumatic reaction. If any type of penetration was involved, they are much more likely to experience severe trauma, which often goes untreated. The abuser's energy and image will often haunt women and show up even when they are safely in the arms of a loving partner. Just like every other pattern and blueprint in our lives, sexual abuse becomes a lasting imprint on women, and they often find themselves moving from one abusive relationship to the next.

For the nervous system to operate at an optimal level, it needs to be in a state of equilibrium, or emotional balance. According to Peter Levine, a leading trauma expert, "trauma is the body's physiological response to an event that overwhelms us, that makes us feel helpless, that makes us feel paralyzed."[6] Trauma disrupts the nervous system and causes it to become dysregulated—usually through over-stimulation. When we become overstimulated, we are typically flooded with fear, anxiety, panic, and rage. We don't know how to deal with this chaotic state and a danger signal goes off in our body. Physiologically, our heart rate and respiration increase as our body starts pumping more adrenaline. We have a hard time processing sensory stimulus since all our attention is focused on the threat. Even our perception of time is impaired. That is why we often hear accident victims say "time slowed down."

Levine studied the response of animals in the wild to understand the human response to trauma. Wild animals are constantly under threat from predators. When attacked by a tiger, its prey either flees to escape the danger or fights to neutralize or fend off the tiger. The animal's nervous system is on high alert signaling "danger." Why then are animals not walking around traumatized? Levine realized that the physical act of fighting or fleeing to escape the danger discharges and releases the trauma. Additionally, violent shaking frequently follows a close call with danger. Shaking is the natural way in which the nervous system comes back into regulation, discharging the trauma. You might have experienced this yourself after an accident, injury, or surgery.

Another response to danger is to freeze. Rather than fight or flee, we physically shut down to preserve our resources. Breathing slows down, digestion stops, and the heart rate decreases. This

6   Peter Levine, *Waking the Tiger: Healing Trauma*. North Atlantic Books, 1997. Print.

shutdown causes numbness, paralysis, and disassociation, which is a sense that you have left your body. In a freeze state, the body is not able to release the trauma, so it gets stuck in the body, causing ongoing dysregulation of the nervous system.

Post-Traumatic Stress Disorder

Unresolved trauma can cause Post-Traumatic Stress Disorder (PTSD), which typically shows up fairly quickly after the traumatic event. Severe PTSD can be quite debilitating. Here are some of the symptoms of PTSD:

- Invasive, disturbing thoughts
- Replaying of the traumatic event
- Severe anxiety
- Insomnia
- Unsettling dreams
- Clinical depression

Individuals who have been sexually abused in childhood typically are plagued with PTSD. The same is true for victims of rape. Trauma can also result from any type of overwhelming experience including physical injuries, surgery, accidents, and life-changing events such as the death of a family member or friend. Whether or not an overwhelming event turns into a trauma or PTSD depends on other circumstances, including one's level of resilience, ability to provide resources to oneself, and whether or not steps are taken after the event to facilitate resolution and healing.

To some extent, who you are as a person and your life experiences will impact how a traumatic event affects you. The more resilient and able to bounce back from adverse events you are, the less likely a traumatic event will have a lasting negative impact. Resilience comes from both your internal and external worlds and your experiences. Individuals who have a sense that the world is a safe place, who do not live in constant chaos or fear for their survival, tend to be more resilient and able to handle traumatic events. They generally know how to care for themselves by taking actions that will help support their well-being and bring them back to a balanced state of mind. This might include reaching out to a friend or therapist, doing meditation or yoga to help calm down, or learning other tools to alleviate trauma.

HOW SEXUAL ABUSE IMPACTS SEXUALITY

The impact of sexual abuse on a woman's sexuality varies greatly. Some common reactions include:

- Physical responses such as painful sex and vaginismus (tightening of the vaginal muscles that prevents penetration)
- Problems experiencing orgasms
- Repression of memories
- Feeling numb when receiving touch
- Becoming easily overwhelmed by sensations and/ or emotions
- Disassociating or leaving the body during sexual activity

Unresolved Trauma Causing Vaginismus: Anne's Story

Mike and Anne had been married for over twenty-six years and had struggled with their sex life throughout their marriage.

Growing up, Anne had been severely abused by a missionary priest while living overseas. Her parents never found out about the abuse, and Anne never resolved the trauma. Like most abuse victims, when Anne reached adulthood, she had a very difficult time setting boundaries because she had been unable to do so with her abuser at a formative age. It's not surprising that her first adult sexual experience was also nonconsensual.

Although she loved her husband, Anne often saw images of the priest when her husband wanted to make love. This retriggered her trauma, causing her whole body to freeze and shut down, including her vagina, which made sex very painful. Anne was experiencing unresolved long-term PTSD. Even the thought of having sex could trigger the memory of her abuser, and her body would react the same way she had during the childhood abuse, recreating a state of "freeze."

Repression of Memories

One common defense mechanism the body uses to protect us is repressing memories. When clients talk about big gaps in their childhood memories, it is often related to some sort of trauma, though not necessarily abuse. In my own case, I had no memories of my childhood from the ages of three to ten until they began to surface in my late forties. My father's death and my mom's subsequent nervous breakdown when I was three were so traumatic that I repressed these memories. I had also buried shameful memories around early childhood sexual exploration, such as the incident with my pet dog. When I began to heal some of my sexual shame by acknowledging these events, other childhood memories also started to come back. While I still don't remember everything about my childhood, I now have a much better understanding of this part of my life.

It's important to know that attempting to dredge up memories of trauma rarely works and often backfires. Trust your body to protect you. The memories will come back when and if you are sufficiently prepared, have the resilience and resources to process them, and can work toward a healing resolution.

Old, unresolved trauma can be healed without accessing your memories at all. Peter Levine has created a very respected approach to trauma therapy called Somatic Experiencing, which he explains in detail in his book *Waking the Tiger*. The premise of this therapy is that wild animals, whose lives are constantly threatened, quickly recover from the traumatic events simply because they release the energy physically by discharging the stress from their bodies, often through uncontrollable shaking. When human beings experience a traumatic event, we override this natural release by bringing in shame, pervasive thoughts, fears, and judgments. Rather than release the trauma, it gets stuck in our body. Somatic Experiencing focuses on releasing the physical aspects of the trauma before dealing with the emotional and cognitive elements.

Trauma and Self-Protection Mechanisms

The body has several ways to "protect" us from the emotional and physical impact of trauma at the actual time of the event. One of the most effective is through the process of disassociation. Disassociation is a detachment from the body, emotions, and memories and a loss of awareness of present circumstances. It can be mild, like when you daydream or get lost in a book. In abuse survivors, it often shows up in a more severe recurrent form during sex.

Trauma and Disassociation: Darla's Story

Darla was struggling with her libido. I quickly noticed that any time Darla started to feel some sensation in her body from my featherlight touch on her arm, she disassociated. She then reported that she felt completely numb when I was touching her. Often women who have been abused will not feel sensation and will completely lose presence. Their partners will report that it looks like they have left their body, and even the room, while having sex. Disassociation is a protective pattern that is learned during abuse. Since the trauma is never resolved, the pattern remains stuck in the body. I worked with Darla to help her create safety in her body and to begin to address the trauma. As the trauma slowly began to release, Darla was able to focus more on sensation and not disassociate.

Trauma and Over-Stimulation: Tonya's Story

Getting overwhelmed by sensation is the flip side of disassociation. It is also caused by not feeling safe in your body. However, instead of leaving the body and numbing out, you become overwhelmed with sensation when the nervous system has been overstimulated. This often leads to anxiety, panic, and fear. Intense deep breathing exercises can trigger this reaction. Unfortunately, I learned this the hard way when I started my practice. I had just hung out my shingle as a sex and intimacy coach when Tonya, a social work student, found me through a Facebook post. She said she was interested in exploring her sexuality, so I scheduled her for a session. While I knew that she had some trauma in her background, I assumed that her social work studies had given her tools and resources that would help her in our work together.

The first lesson I learned: never assume anything! As was my practice at the time, I had Tonya do some deep belly breathing to help her relax and gain access to sensation. Thirty minutes into our session, it was clear that Tonya was having a traumatic response. She was breathing heavily, her skin was clammy, she was agitated, and her eyes were glazed over in fear. This was the opposite reaction from what I anticipated, so I directed her to return to normal breathing and come back to her body in present time. Deep breathing can create sensations in the body, which is generally a good thing. In Tonya's case, the sensations overwhelmed her, and her nervous system became dysregulated. The second lesson I learned: never start a new client with deep breathing exercises. I learned to start slowly and teach them some breathing exercises to quiet the nervous system during the early exploration stage.

Slaying the Tiger: Ellen's Story

Not every woman who has experienced abuse has long-lasting trauma. Sometimes we are able to process and discharge the trauma fairly immediately, as a tiger does in the wild, or by resolving the trauma in some other way that arises on its own. Ellen is the perfect example. At the age of seven, Ellen and her younger brother befriended a teenage boy. During a game of hide and seek, the teenager grabbed Ellen, pulled down his pants, and made her suck him. Overpowered by his physical strength and silenced by his threat to tell her parents, Ellen complied with his demand. She did not tell anyone about what had happened. For months after the abuse, Ellen had a recurring dream of this incident. Normally this is a sign of PTSD, but in this case, Ellen was able to process her trauma in the dream by escaping from the teenager without being abused. The escape varied from dream to dream from shouting for help to kicking him in the balls. During the real event, she was in a freeze state. But in her dreams, she moved into a fight-or-flight response, which allowed the trauma to be released from her body and her psyche.

Downstream Effects of Abuse

Trauma and Fear of Intimacy: Lilly's Story

For most women, sexual abuse creates fear of intimacy, which makes it challenging for them to trust men. Survivors of abuse are often experts at creating barriers to keep others at a safe distance. Meet Lilly and Matt, married for five years and struggling with their sex life. Lilly complained that she was no longer attracted to Matt, but Matt still adored her. Following a history of severe childhood abuse, Lilly had been sexually open prior to marriage. She'd slept with lots of men and had been attracted to the bad boys who treated her poorly and abused her. Matt was anything but a bad boy. He was a tenured professor and a stable and loving presence in Lilly's life, something she needed desperately. But Lilly had never been sexually attracted to Matt. She did not like the way he smelled and cringed every time he touched her.

Matt tried everything. He cleaned up his diet and used special soaps and deodorants, but nothing covered up the scent of his natural pheromones. Lilly continued to be repelled by his smell. She'd been drawn to Matt because he was the good boy. She knew he would provide for her and fulfill her need for a loving and supportive home. Lilly also knew at an unconscious level that if she was not sexually attracted to Matt, she could hold intimacy at bay. Her reaction to his smell and touch was her way of putting up barriers to intimacy. Matt was willing to put in the work, but Lilly was not, and they ultimately separated.

Harming and otherwise abusing oneself is another common reaction to sexual abuse caused by low self-esteem and feelings of worthlessness. For some women, self-abuse involves cutting themselves or taking risks in order to actually feel sensation in their body. Extremely promiscuous behavior is also a form of self-harm. One client told me that she'd had sex with over two hundred men but had never had a satisfying relationship.

Trauma and Self-Abusive Behavior: Cecilia's Story

Cecilia and Brad were referred to me by a physical therapist to help resolve her vaginismus. In her twenties, Cecilia had hundreds of one-night stands, struggled with alcohol and drug addiction, and abused her body. She even became a sex worker for a few years. This was part of her healing path, since as a sex worker, she was able to set and maintain her boundaries and control who she had sex with. During this time, she met Brad. He was the first man who loved and respected her. Cecilia's vaginismus started three months after they got engaged.

There was nothing physically wrong with Cecilia. Her vaginismus was a self-protective mechanism that blocked her from true intimacy with Brad. For Celia, sex and love were not connected. As her feelings for Brad grew, it became harder for her to separate the two, so her body did that for her, and by so doing kept her safe from exploring intimacy. Luckily for Celia, Brad was totally invested in the relationship. We worked together as a partnership, with Brad becoming Celia's sexual healer while I helped her resolve her trauma and intimacy blocks.

MEN AND SEXUAL TRAUMA

Many men have also experienced sexual abuse at the hands of men or women. One in six boys has been abused before the age of eighteen, according to a 2005 study by the US Centers for Disease Control. It is likely these incidents are significantly underreported, especially when the definition of rape is changed to include being forced to penetrate. Men who are abused by a parent or close relative have severe psychological damage. Common effects on men include:

- Anger management issues
- Anxiety and fear
- Confusion over sexual orientation (when abused by a man)
- Feelings of helplessness and depression
- Fear of intimacy
- Sexual dysfunction

Recreating Abusive Relationships: David's Story

Men who have been abused by their mothers tend to have major issues with trust and intimacy. Like women who are abused, they tend to recreate the abusive relationship. David is a recently divorced thirty-five-year-old CEO of a successful software company. After separating from his wife, he began having dreams about his childhood, and then memories of being abused by his mother began to surface in his awareness. From age seven to twelve, she'd made him stroke her naked body. For David, this was the only time that he felt close to and comforted by his mother, who otherwise ignored him, no matter how hard he tried to please her. No surprise then that he married an emotionally abusive, cold and distant, sexually selfish woman whom he was also unable to please.

David started seeing me when he separated from his ex-wife. He had recreated the habit from his childhood of incessantly touching women whom he was dating, even in his sleep. Initiating sex was extremely challenging for David. He was attracted to domineering women who then complained when he was too passive during sex.

When David first came to me for therapy, he simply could not receive pleasure from a woman. When I touched him during a session, he would completely disassociate. Over several years, David learned that it was safe to receive pleasure, regained his sexual confidence, and had healthy intimate relationships with women.

If you have experienced severe sexual abuse or trauma, the road to healing and sexual awakening can be fraught with danger, so you would do well to work with a qualified practitioner who is experienced with working with trauma. I have witnessed far too many abuse survivors who get enticed to join "sex-positive" communities and programs that are not appropriately staffed with coaches and practitioners qualified to work with trauma. This is a major oversight, given the fact that one in four women and one in six men have experienced sexual abuse. The boundaries in some of these programs are fuzzy, which creates further problems for boundary-challenged sexual abuse survivors, and can at times reawaken old traumas.

Working with Sexual Trauma

Slow and gentle is the best approach for clients with sexual abuse, unless they have done a significant amount of recovery work and are extremely well-resourced. Trying to address your sexual issues if you have not first addressed your trauma is ineffective and will often make matters even worse. My approach to working through trauma is drawn from body-based modalities such as Somatic Experiencing. We focus on helping to rewire the nervous system after trauma and release the ingrained fight, flight, and freeze responses when the body senses danger.

Above all, individuals with sexual abuse issues need to feel safe both within their bodies and in their external environment. Feeling safe within one's body can be challenging and scary. Depending on your level of resilience and your ability to care for yourself and transform the way in which your nervous system reacted to the abuse, it can take a significant period of time to establish safety in the body. Once safety is established, we work on creating and honoring boundaries, since abuse victims almost always have difficulty with boundaries. Over time, we begin specific practices that allow the trauma to be released from the body, creating more capacity to experience sensation and pleasure.

Resolving Trauma and Reclaiming Their Sex Life: Jessie and Mark's Story

Jessie and Mark came to see me because Jessie often lost her desire for sex or just shut down in the middle of it for no obvious reason. They were both frustrated by this and wanted me to help them "find their sexy." As a couple, they were very involved in the sex-positive community, attended many workshops and trainings, and regularly made use of several sexual practices drawn from different schools. Despite this, they were still struggling in their sex life.

Jessie had been sexually abused as a child, but she had never done specific work around the abuse. She struggled with a lack of sensation in her body and disassociation during sex, a common experience of survivors of trauma. She wasn't ready to address the trauma, so we worked on intimacy exercises. In one session, Jessie and Mark were touching each other and building up erotic energy. Jessie said that she was feeling turned on by Mark, which was unusual for her. I watched her arousal increase, and then in a blink of an eye, it completely disappeared. She had a blank look on her face, and no matter what I suggested, Jessie could not find her arousal again.

Jessie said this was very common and often happened to her during sex. It was clear to me that Jessie's disassociation was due to her unresolved trauma, and I strongly suggested that she work on healing it. But Jessie was not ready. However, after several months without any marked improvement in their sex life, Jesse finally agreed to do some trauma work, and I met with her individually on a weekly basis. Within a few months, she began to feel sensations in her body as some of the old trauma was released. Jessie's body became a safe, rather than unsafe, place to be. Once this safety was established, her libido improved. She began to recognize signs of disassociation, and she had tools at her disposal to prevent her from feeling unsafe. Then we were able to successfully address the sexual issues in the relationship, which also improved dramatically.

In the next chapter, we will learn how physical injuries from accidents, surgeries, and childbirth can also cause wounding around our sexuality. All of these impede our ability to live an orgasmic life.

Chapter 6

THE BODY REMEMBERS: TRAUMA & PHYSICAL IMPRINTING

Trauma and Physical Imprinting

Sexual trauma does not just happen from sexual abuse. Remember that trauma can be the result of any event that overwhelms us and makes us feel helpless. We can be traumatized by an accident, surgery, injury, medical procedure, or chronic health condition. Any one of these events can impact our sexuality even though the bodily harm wasn't directly related to sexual activity. Physical trauma that affects your sexuality happens quite frequently, although it tends not to be acknowledged. Like any type of trauma, this can also have a huge impact on our emotional well-being.

What makes this trauma particularly challenging is that even though the actual physical wound or injury may heal, the imprint of that wound on our body can remain for decades. Bessel van der Kolk, a pioneer in the trauma field, talks about cellular memory in his book, *The Body Keeps the Score: Brain, Mind, and Body in the Healing of Trauma.* Cellular memory means that from a somatic perspective, the body remembers every type of experience we've ever had. Visualize your body as the hard drive of a computer.

Everything that has ever happened to you is recorded in the cells of your body, similarly to files being stored within a computer.

The relatively new field of epigenetics takes this theory even further. Epigenetics is the concept that people are impacted by environmental factors such as diet, lifestyle choices, behavior, and trauma, and that those influences can be passed on to their descendants as genetic modification. Evidence of this has shown up in children and grandchildren of Holocaust survivors. When examining cortisol levels (the stress hormone that helps the body return to normal after trauma), these Holocaust descendants were found to have significantly lower levels of cortisol in their bodies than in the general population. Low cortisol levels are common for those who suffer from PTSD. Thus, the Holocaust descendants were born with the genetic markers for trauma.[7]

Body Memory

Body memory theory states that the process of storing memories happens not just in the brain, but in the actual physical body itself. Here's an example of how it works.

Imagine that as a child, you were a good ice skater, but you haven't put on ice skates in decades. You're invited to go ice-skating and feel a little nervous about how you will perform. Will you be smooth or will you fall, and will it feel awkward? Within minutes of getting out on the ice, you're skating freely, as if you had never stopped. Why? Body memory. Your body remembers not only how to skate, it remembers the freedom, agility, and confidence you felt on the ice. Compare this to someone who was a bad ice skater, someone who felt awkward, lost their balance

---

7   Bessel van der Kolk, *The Body Keeps the Score: Brain, Mind and Body in the Healing of Trauma*. Penguin Books, Reprint Edition, Sept 2015. Print.

and fell a lot, and was afraid of being hurt. When this person puts on skates and gets on the ice, all of their body memories activate. They tense up, go slowly and cautiously, and feel anxious rather than confident and free.

This same type of body memory experience plays itself out when we experience physical wounding around our sexuality. My body shut down sexually because of a series of physical wounds in my teens and twenties. I lost my virginity when I was sixteen to my high school boyfriend, and rather than having tears of joy roll down my cheeks, I sobbed in pain. The pain I felt from sex that day was burned into me as a body memory, and it lived on in my body for thirty-five years. Unfortunately, it is not uncommon for women to experience sex as painful. More than 25 percent of women experience vaginismus, i.e., ongoing pain with intercourse. Over 80 percent have experienced painful sex at some point in their lives. This often occurs during periods of hormonal change such as the postpartum period and menopause.

Looking back, I now realize that my negative relationship with my vagina started when I was eleven years old and had painful and heavy periods. They made me hate everything having to do with my reproductive organs. The shame associated with period accidents made me hate my vagina even more. When I found out that sex was painful and not pleasurable, I was furious with my vagina for letting me down once again. At the time, I didn't realize that the fear of having painful sex would quickly become its own self-fulfilling prophecy. My anxiety about feeling pain caused my vagina to tighten up to the point that I was unable to relax and enjoy foreplay. Oral sex was also not enjoyable because of fear and anxiety related to the experience with my pet dog. No surprise then that orgasms were totally elusive. Since I couldn't get aroused, pain-free intercourse was not possible.

I felt like a broken woman and believed my body simply wasn't built for sex. I put up with a lot of painful sex, hoping it would be different, and that I could experience pleasure during lovemaking, but I never did. Sex also led to recurring bladder and yeast infections requiring doctor's visits. My body was further traumatized by excruciating procedures at the hands of urologists trying to dilate the urethral canal to help prevent chronic bladder infections. Daily doses of antibiotics just exacerbated my yeast infections.

Is it any wonder that my body just shut down sexually and that it posted a "Closed for Business" sign after my second child was born? My body associated sex with pain, discomfort, medications, and medical procedures—nowhere in my body memory had sex been a source of pleasure. This was hardly the stuff of romance novels or passionate nights of lovemaking.

Physical Trauma's Impact on Sexuality

Physical trauma from medical procedures is quite common among women. Caesarean sections, hysterectomies, breast surgeries, and urinary tract surgeries are all culprits. Episiotomies, a common procedure that women experience during childbirth, result in scar tissue around the perineum that causes pain during intercourse. Indeed, any type of surgery or medical procedure can cause trauma to the body. The body typically heals itself, so most women's sex lives are not affected long-term by these experiences. But for some women, the impact on their sex life can be quite significant.

Physical trauma also has an emotional component. While physical wounds heal, the emotional impact of the experience and the trauma the body went through remains with us until and unless we release it. The cellular memory of the trauma lives on in the parts of our bodies that have been wounded. Women routinely break down in tears when I touch or honor the manifestation of their physical wounds: the scar from the C-section, reconstructed breasts after a mastectomy, the empty womb space after the hysterectomy, or the third or fourth degree episiotomy scars.

MEN ALSO EXPERIENCE PHYSICAL TRAUMA THAT AFFECTS THEIR SEXUALITY

Vasectomies, penile implants, hernia operations, prostate cancer, and testicular cancer can cause physical as well as emotional wounding. Often the cock shuts down, and men struggle with getting an erection. Sometimes this is physiological, particularly in the case of prostate surgery, but very often there is an emotional component. Men feel like they've lost their virility, their ego is bruised, or they begin to face their own mortality.

Circumcision is a very common physical trauma, especially when done without anesthesia. There is a growing recognition in medicine and psychology that routine circumcision needs to be reconsidered and that trauma from circumcision can have long-term negative psychological effects. A male colleague who is also a trauma specialist helps men resolve circumcision trauma. These men often experience difficulty getting and maintaining an erection, and some are troubled by delayed ejaculation due to reduced sensitivity. More times than not, the minute my colleague touches these men anywhere near their penises, they start clenching their hands like a baby does when distressed. Circumcision is the perfect setup for trauma. An infant is strapped down, insufficiently anesthetized, and the extremely sensitive tissue of his sex organ is cut. This immediately puts the body into a freeze state. The baby is helpless and overwhelmed with fear and pain. Often these memories are deeply repressed, but when sexual issues start occurring, this deep wounding and trauma can come to light.

Heal the Body, Heal the Mind

The more I work with the human body, the more in awe I am of our body's connection to our emotions, experiences, and states of being. Your body is a memory bank for every significant experience in your life. These memories lie deep within your organs, muscles, nervous system, and the emotional centers in your body.

Eastern medicine and philosophy take a holistic approach to healing, connecting our physical body with our emotions. The ancient practices of Taoism, Tantra, and Chinese medicine align our emotional, physical, and energetic bodies. This alignment is an important step toward living an orgasmic life. It recognizes the flow between our emotions, our physical bodies, and our energy. If even one of them is blocked, the connection is also disrupted and we cannot be in flow. Western medicine is slowly catching up with this approach by creating medical specialties in Mind-Body Medicine. Meditation, acupuncture, and some forms of energy healing are becoming more mainstream. Research studies demonstrating the health benefits of meditation and acupuncture are validating what eastern medicine has known all along: our emotions impact our physical health and well-being.

Over the last decade, the National Center for Comprehensive and Integrative Health has funded a series of mindfulness studies that demonstrate meditation's positive effects on anxiety, depression, pain, smoking cessation, high blood pressure, supportive treatment for cancer, sleep disturbances, and symptoms of menopause. Brain scans of meditators show functional differences, including changes in brain volume in four areas: focus, memory and cognition, empathy and compassion, and emotional regulation. Studies on the effectiveness of acupuncture show significant health benefits in the treatment of pain and headaches and as a supportive therapy for cancer patients.

Likewise, the field of somatic psychology views the mind and body as an integrated whole. From this perspective, healing is most effective when the physical and psychological wounds are addressed at the same time. We cannot heal the mind without healing the body, and we can't heal the body without healing the mind. I hold this truth deep in my heart, having witnessed it over and over in my life and in the lives of my clients.

For this very reason, I was drawn to Tantra and sacred sexuality. When I recognized the connection between my sexual problems and the feelings of anxiety and fear that tracked back to the incident with my pet dog, I realized that I had so much shame and anxiety from that experience that my vagina started to contract whenever I felt aroused. This occurred anytime I wanted to have sex, causing pain and discomfort during penetration. It took me decades to realize that the recurring vaginal and urinary tract infections were also related to my fear.

In Chinese medicine the five organ systems—liver, kidney, heart, lung, and spleen—are associated with five emotions: anger, sadness, happiness, fear, and anxiety. Fear is the prevalent emotion for the kidney system, which includes the bladder, kidneys, and reproductive organs. Fear causes pain and disease in the kidneys and adrenals, creating the perfect environment for UTIs and vaginal infections. Anxiety has the most impact on the spleen, which includes the stomach. Not surprisingly, I had chronic digestive troubles: irritable bowel syndrome, gastrointestinal reflux, and constipation.

Releasing Trapped Pain
from Trauma

Physical trauma in the body is caused by an endless cycle of pain and fear that feeds on itself. My initial fear about painful intercourse turned into the fear that sex would land me in the urologist's office, where I would undergo painful procedures. I became more anxious every time this occurred, and my fear of sex was heightened. No wonder my body froze and my vagina closed up with the possibility of any penetration. It's impossible to relax and enjoy sex when anxiety and fear consume you.

The fear/pain cycle very frequently occurs as a result of physical injuries and can be quite debilitating. If you have ever had chronic muscle pain (back, neck, hip, shoulder) attributed to a physical activity, you have likely experienced that cycle. Say you "pull your back" lifting something heavy and are out of commission for a period of time. Each time you lift something heavy thereafter, your body reacts in fear. This causes the muscles to contract, and the stress that results can bring on muscle spasms and thereby increase the fear associated with lifting.

A similar cycle occurs for those who have experienced sexual abuse or sexual trauma. Your body associates sex with an emotion or a past painful or traumatic event. In my case, my body associated sex with fear and pain. Abuse survivors may associate sex with a variety of emotions, including fear, anger, disgust, shame, and even guilt. This is especially true if they felt aroused or had an orgasm during the abuse—both normal physiological responses to sexual stimulation, regardless of whether the stimulation is welcome or not. All of these emotions can cause the body to contract and shut down. Each also feeds on itself, creating a vicious cycle that is hard to break.

SOME OF THE SEXUAL PROBLEMS THAT CAN OCCUR FROM PHYSICAL TRAUMA INCLUDE:

- Lack of arousal
- Numbing of bodily sensations
- Difficulty achieving orgasm
- Freezing or disassociating
- Vaginismus and painful sex
- Erection issues

Trauma from a Routine Gynecological Exam: Raina's Story

Raina and her husband wanted to get pregnant, but severe vaginismus made sex extremely painful. When he would attempt to penetrate her, she felt as if knives were ripping her skin. Her husband couldn't even get a finger inside her. Raina's OB/GYN said there was nothing physically wrong and gave her dilators to stretch her vagina. The dilators were painful and did not work. She'd grown up in a sexually repressed environment, and there was no evidence of abuse. Her family was from India, and as prescribed by their cultural beliefs, she was a virgin until she married. But none of this accounts for the fact that she was completely disconnected from her sexuality. What had happened to her pussy to cause so much pain with penetration?

Like so many women, Raina had experienced trauma during a gynecological exam. This is more common than you might think. At her first pelvic exam, Raina was still a virgin and was nervous. Her anxiety was compounded by a friend who told her the exam would be painful. Raina's body was tense before she went into the examining room. When the doctor inserted the speculum into her vagina, she practically jumped off the table in pain. Thus began her body's attempt to protect her pussy from penetration. Her body shut down and her vagina closed up. This initiated her pain/fear cycle.

Raina had heard that sex was pleasurable, but that was not her experience. Instead of relaxing during sex, her whole body would contract as she braced against the pain of penetration. During one of our bodywork sessions, after she was completely relaxed and highly aroused, she experienced pain-free finger penetration. For the first time ever, her vagina started to feel pleasure rather than pain. This helped to break the pain/fear cycle. Raina is now pregnant with her second child.

Holistic Pelvic Care

Holistic Pelvic Care™ is a specialized practice that alleviates congestion in the pelvic bowl to restore balance on energetic, physical, and emotional levels. Founded by Tami Lynn Kent, a physical therapist and energy healer, Holistic Pelvic Care recognizes that a woman's pelvic bowl "root" contains a vast array of information and that it is an access point to emotions, traumatic events in our lives, and our connection with spirit. Congestion in the pelvic bowl blocks the flow of energy in the body. These blocks take many forms, from unexpressed emotions such as grief and anger, to physical wounds from surgeries and childbirth, to sexual abuse and trauma. Holistic Pelvic Care is extremely useful for postpartum women and helps to restore tissue damage from childbirth as well as strengthen the pelvic floor muscles.

Trauma from childbirth, while not often discussed, can significantly impact our sexuality. Left untreated, childbirth trauma can live on in the body for years or even decades after the birth. Giving birth in itself causes trauma to the body, just like any other intense physical and emotional experience. But trauma from childbirth can also happen during labor and delivery, particularly if things do not go according to plan. I often see this resulting from unplanned C-sections, complicated labor and deliveries, and in cases of fetal distress when the baby is rushed to the ICU. Second and third-degree vaginal tears during birth, episiotomies, and subsequent internal stitches can also cause physical and emotional trauma for the new mom.

Healing Childbirth Trauma: Carrie's Story

Carrie came to see me six months postpartum for a Holistic Pelvic Care session because she was shut down sexually and disconnected from her body. Carrie had been a very sexually open woman before and during her pregnancy but had completely lost her libido after the birth. As we got into our session, Carrie told me that despite having had a difficult forty-eight-hour labor, she had made it very clear to her husband and her medical team that she did not want a C-section. Against her objections, her medical team deemed a C-section necessary, and she appealed to her husband for some more time to try to deliver vaginally. He did not support her decision, so Carrie agreed to the C-section. Complications ensued, and Carrie had a transfusion and a long recovery. She did not feel like herself for many months and did not enjoy motherhood as much as she'd expected.

The childbirth was traumatic for Carrie in many ways. Besides the physical trauma to her body from the surgery, Carrie also carried emotional trauma. She had felt completely out of control during the birth and had felt betrayed by her body, her medical team, and her husband. On an intellectual level, she knew the C-section had been a medical necessity, but nonetheless, she was left with a deep emotional wound. She had not been able to access or process the trauma, so it remained in her body. Naturally, she felt disconnected from her body and sexuality. The anger and resentment she was harboring toward her husband also zapped her libido.

Fortunately, Carrie reached out for help, and with coaching and Holistic Pelvic Care, she released the trauma, processed her anger, and rekindled her sex life in a relatively short period of time.

I consider a woman's pelvic bowl (uterus, ovaries, vagina) to be her second heart and second brain—the source of tremendous love and wisdom and the gateway to orgasmic life energy. It is from this place of birth and rebirth that we sow the seeds for all our future endeavors and deeply connect to all our emotions, including those in the deep recesses of our brain and our body. Later in this book, you will have an opportunity to listen to the voice of your own pelvic bowl.

In Taoist sexual practices and reflexology, the cervix, the opening to the uterus, is the heart point in women. Stimulating it brings up a range of emotions. The uterus also holds all of our wounding, both physical and emotional. Activation from penetration or any type of touch—physical or energetic—can trigger these wounds. If you've ever cried during sex for no particular reason, it's likely that you are releasing some blocked emotions or trauma. I always tell men not to take it personally if a woman cries during sex because there's a 95 percent chance that it has nothing to do with them.

Weaning Herself Off a Vibrator: Jane's Story

Jane came to me with a common problem among women: she could only have a clitoral orgasm with a vibrator. As with those who use a vibrator on a regular basis, her clitoris became de-sensitized. Jane's clitoris became accustomed to stimulation that was fast, hard, and strong, unlike any that can be performed with a finger or a tongue. Electrically powered stimulation was the only way Jane could climax; anything less did not give her sufficient arousal. (Similarly, some men can only orgasm during masturbation with a particular stroke; fast, hard, and strong.)

The good news is that your body is extremely intelligent. Information to the brain is relayed from nerve endings throughout the body via neural pathways. Your body can form new neural pathways through a process known as neuroplasticity wherein the brain starts linking neurons together in new ways. The brain does this automatically every time you learn something new. Once new neural pathways are activated, you can change unwanted patterns stuck in the body. Hands-on Sexological Bodywork is one of the most effective ways to create new neural pathways of sensation and pleasure. This sex education modality helps clients connect with their sexuality through one-way touch from practitioner to client. Once Jane learned new ways to stroke her clitoris and touch her vulva, she was able to wean herself off the vibrator.

We all can rewire our brain to experience new sensations and pleasure pathways and embody the erotic aspect of who we are as human beings. You have to be open to trying new ways of receiving touch and pleasure and be patient, however, because neuroplasticity does not happen overnight. This next exercise will help you create new neural pathways on your lips.

Exercise: Awakening New Pleasure Pathways

This exercise will take three to five minutes. Find a quiet space. Close your eyes, feel your feet on the ground, and take a long, deep breath. Notice the lips on your mouth. Without touching them, begin to visualize how you would like to touch your lips with one finger to feel pleasure. Then physically do that. Notice if what you imagined actually feels good. Repeat this action ten times, and notice how much or how little sensation and pleasure you experience. You will probably notice the sensation and pleasure decreasing at some point. Your lips might go numb, or you might start to feel annoyed by the touch. All of these are normal and good things to observe about your experience. Now let's create some new pleasure pathways. Try all of these or come up with your own:

- Run your finger around your lips very slowly and lightly
- Use your fingernail to touch your lips
- Gently tap your lips, making sure not to miss any spots
- Using one finger, gently and slowly pull your lower lip forward as if you were strumming a guitar string
- Run your tongue around your lips
- Find a soft object (shirt sleeve, scarf, feather, etc.) and run that object around your lips

Notice all the new ways you can experience pleasure and sensation on your lips. If you want to be really adventurous, do this same exercise, by yourself or with a partner, on your pussy. You will be surprised at how many different ways you can experience pleasure just by varying the type and speed of touch.

New pathways to experience sensation and pleasure are always available and will make your sex life more fun and juicy, but most of us don't even know they exist. One of the reasons that women complain about not being turned on is because their partner touches them the exact same way every time they have sex. Touch that is predictable or repetitive loses the sexual charge it had when it was new and exciting. Dulled nerves might even make it feel numb or annoying. The solution to this problem is to explore new ways in which you can experience pleasure and different bodily sensations. This creates new pathways of pleasure in your body, heightening sensation because it is a different pattern.

Activating New Pleasure Pathways: Ingrid and Mark's Story

Ingrid and Mark were newlyweds struggling in the bedroom. Determined to improve his skills, Mark took a workshop on G-spot stimulation. He loved his workshop partner's response and really wanted Ingrid to have this experience. Ingrid was willing, but when Mark touched her G-spot, she either felt nothing or experienced discomfort. Mark blamed himself, thinking, "I must be a bad student…it must be my technique. How am I ever going to be a good lover?" This made him wary of trying anything new. It wasn't long before their sex life fell apart.

Ingrid and Mark were open to receiving hands-on instruction on G-spot massage with Ingrid as our model. Mark's technique was great, but Ingrid still felt nothing. She was frustrated with her lack of sensation and made Mark stop after just a few minutes. This was part of the problem. Neither of them understood that nerve endings in the G-spot need to be activated to create a new pleasure pathway, and that takes time. I coached Ingrid to be patient with herself and with her husband. I showed Mark how to use gentle stimulation while Ingrid put her entire focus on receiving sensation. Their homework was to go home and play. Ingrid paid close attention, and as instructed, was patient while Mark gently explored her vagina and found her G-spot. The initial discomfort she felt at his touch gave way to pleasure in short order. Many a women has this exact experience when a lover focuses on her G-spot. Discomfort in the G-spot is often unreleased emotional pain. Once that block is removed, there is more room for pleasure.

Now that you have a better understanding of the impact of shame, sexual abuse, physical wounding, and trauma on our connection with our sexuality, we are going to turn our attention in Chapter 7 to blocks around intimacy, which are also a product of our upbringing and sexual blueprint.

Chapter 7

BLOCKS TO INTIMACY

Our desire for intimacy with another human being is a basic human need. We are born completely helpless, "little blobs of protoplasm" as my ex-husband fondly called our infant sons. Without human support to meet our needs for food and shelter, we would quickly die. But infants need more than food and shelter to thrive. They need a strong attachment with a primary caregiver. This attachment sets up key conditions that allow for healthy intimate relationships. Likewise, a lack of attachment predisposes us to difficulty in this crucial area of our lives.

Attachment Theory ("It really is all your mother's fault")

Attachment theory, which originates in research by developmental psychologist John Bowlby and Mary Ainsworth in the 1960s and '70s, tells us that children will have different patterns of attachment depending primarily on how they experienced their early caregiving environment. Early patterns of attachment shape, but do not determine, the individual's expectations in later relationships. Attachment theory identifies four distinct attachment styles. According to Bowlby, a child's attachment style results from the caregiver's behavior. It is essentially the way any individual child responds to the adult they interact with the most.

Childhood Attachment Styles, John Bowlby, 1969

Attachment Styles	% of sample (also generalized to represent US population	The child's general state of being	Mother's responsiveness to her child's signals and needs	Fullfillment of the child's needs (why the child acts the way it does)
Secure Attachment	65%	• Secure • Explorative • Happy	• Quick • Sensitive • Consistent	Believes and truts that his/her needs will be met
Avoidant Attachment	20%	• Not very explorative • Emotionally distant	• Distant • Disengaged	Subconsciously believes that his/her needs probably won't be met
Ambivalent Attachment	10-15%	• Anxious • Insecure • Angry	• Inconsistent • Sometimes sensitive • Sometimes neglectful	Cannot rely on his/her needs being met
Anxious Avoidant Attachment	10-15%	• Deppressed • Angry • Completely passive • Nonresponsive	• Extreme • Erratic • Frightened or frightening • Passive or intrusive	Severly confused

- Securely attached children: Caregiver responds to child's needs, reacts quickly and positively
- Anxiously attached children: Caregiver responds to child's needs inconsistently
- Avoidantly attached children: Caregiver is unresponsive, uncaring, dismissive
- Anxious Avoidant or Disorganized: Caregiver is abusive or neglectful, responds in frightening ways

These attachment styles follow us into our adult life. In their groundbreaking book, _Attached_, authors Amir Levine and Rachel Heller explain the science of adult attachment and how it impacts our ability to form healthy relationships. According to Levine and Heller, secure people feel comfortable with intimacy and are usually warm and loving, anxious people crave intimacy, are often preoccupied with their relationships, and tend to worry about their partner's ability to love them back, and avoidant people equate intimacy with a loss of independence and constantly try to minimize closeness. Additionally, some people flip back and forth between anxious and avoidant attachment styles.

Adult attachment styles impact:

- Our view of intimacy and togetherness
- The way we deal with conflicts
- Our attitude toward sex
- Our ability to communicate our wishes and needs
- Our expectations for our partner and our relationship[8]

Let's take a little deeper dive into these attachment styles, since they have a significant impact on your ability to create intimacy. As you read through these descriptions, notice which resonates the most with you. This will give you some indication about your own attachment style. You can find any number of tests to evaluate your attachment style online. I highly recommend the one Levine and Heller present in their book. You can find it here: www.attachedthebook.com

---

8   Amir Levine and Rachel Heller, _Attached: The New Science of Adult Attachment and How it can Help You Find and Keep Love._ TarcherPerigree, 2010. Print.

Secure Attachment

A secure attachment style is the best predictor of happy and healthy relationships. This is what we all strive for. If you are secure, you are consistent, reliable, and not afraid of intimacy. You can communicate your needs and desires and easily respond to your partner's needs. You are not prone to "playing games," can help diffuse conflict, are forgiving, and tend to view sex and emotional intimacy as one. "No drama" is your criteria for a healthy relationship.

Anxious Attachment

If you have an anxious attachment style you crave intimacy, but are oversensitive to the moods and fluctuations of your partner. You fear losing them and often act out. Sometimes this shows up as being clingy or needy, which can actually drive them away. You are always waiting for the "other shoe to drop" and have a hard time trusting your partner.

Avoidant Attachment

Deep down, those with an avoidant attachment style want connection and intimacy. However, the need for sovereignty and independence always rules the day. If you have an avoidant style, you are uncomfortable with too much intimacy and closeness. You are emotionally shut down, avoid conflict with a partner by "disappearing," and are constantly taking actions to drive your partner away.

Anxious Avoidant Attachment

A small percentage of people, including me, have an anxious avoidant attachment style. This is the worst of both worlds as your behavior flips back and forth between anxious and avoidant. If someone starts getting too close to you, you push them away. But then once there is some distance, you become anxious that they don't love you and become needy and clingy.

Other Influences on Attachment

Attachment styles are not solely dependent on early experiences with caregivers. Other events can also impact our attachment styles. For example, even those of us who were securely attached as infants can become anxious or avoidant if we experience trauma or if key relationships in childhood are disrupted. This was my situation. I had a secure attachment to both my parents; my father and I were especially close. From the stories I have been told, I was the apple of his eye. My dad was the one who held and nurtured me, while my mother, who was never the touchy-feely type, frequently put her own needs before those of her children. Her own anxious attachment style caused a lot of pain and attachment wounds for my oldest brother, who is sixteen years my senior. When he was just eighteen months old, she sent him away to stay with a relative so she could live with my father, who was stationed in Mississippi during the Korean War.

My dad suddenly died of a massive heart attack when I had just turned three. My life was turned upside down. I had lost my father, and with him, the secure attachment that I needed to thrive. In response to his death, my mother had a nervous breakdown that put her out of commission for over a year. My aunt and my grandmother came to live with us for a time, but my grandmother was not the nurturing type, and I never felt comfortable around her. My oldest brother had already moved out of the house. My other brother, thirteen years older than I was, did his best to step into my dad's shoes as the man of the house and the father figure. But that was a lot to ask of a sixteen-year-old who was deep in his own grief.

Luckily, we lived in a real neighborhood, on a block where everyone knew each other. We all went to the same synagogue, and the kids grew up together. I had a myriad of "aunts and uncles" whose houses I could visit who would feed me and play with me, and who even took me to the bagel store every Sunday morning, just like my dad used to do. It was helpful to have this supportive network and to know that I was loved and cared for. Still, the child in me still felt like I had been abandoned, not only by my father, but also by my mother. Even as my mother got back on her feet, she was emotionally unstable and very needy. No surprise then that I was a highly anxious child who spent a lot of time huddled under my covers with my favorite blanket and my thumb!

Then, when I was eight, my world once again came crashing down. My brother, who had been living with us during college and serving as a surrogate father figure, left for medical school. At the same time, my mom decided to sell our family home and move to a nearby town. All of this separation, both from my neighborhood "aunts and uncles" and from my brother, put me over the edge. I dropped into a deep depression and spent the better part of my days in the school psychologist's office.

Just like we have a sexual blueprint, we also have a blueprint for intimacy based on our attachment styles and early childhood experience. My father's sudden death took me from being securely attached to being anxiously avoidant. My anxious style made separation and loss very hard for me. When I was sent to sleep-away camp at age ten, I was so homesick that I cried myself to sleep every night. At the same time, my avoidant style made me very self-reliant, because I could not rely on my mother to take care of me emotionally. This also made it quite difficult for me to confide in my mother or even make friends among my peers.

As an adult, this intimacy blueprint had a significant impact on my relationships with men. While I desperately desired closeness with my husband, I was unable to open up to him. I struggled to feel and connect with my emotions. Most of the time I was emotionally numb. Occasionally I would feel some sadness, and then I would go immediately into overwhelm, which made me shut down my emotions again. I struggled to feel empathy for my husband, who like my mother, needed a tremendous amount of emotional support.

My deep-seated fear of being alone led me to stay in my dysfunctional marriage for ten years beyond the point where it was clearly over and not serving either one of us. Coupled with this was the lesson that my widowed mother taught me about love, which took me decades to actually understand. She grieved for my father till the day she died, and never remarried or dated another man. From her example, I learned to equate love with grief and pain. So naturally, I chose to marry a man who was in deep grief and pain over the tragic death of his older sister. My job was to fix him, just as I had tried to fix my mother's grief. Not surprisingly, I repeated this pattern with my first post-divorce relationship and ended up with an emotionally abusive man. It wasn't until I got into my first healthy relationship did I realize that love can equal joy. What a relief that was!

The Influence of Attachment Styles in Adult Relationships

Attachment issues tend to repeat themselves from relationship to relationship. I see this again and again with my clients. While everyone struggles with intimacy, it seems to be more prevalent in men. The most common complaint I hear from my female clients who are struggling with their marriage is that they want more intimacy. Intimacy is about expressing your emotions, a basic human function that is socialized out of men. When a little girl falls down on the playground and starts crying, her parents will go to her, let her cry, hold her, and comfort her. But when a little boy falls down, the most common response is to tell him, "Don't cry, you're fine," and send him on his way. Boys rarely see their fathers become emotional or cry, so they have no male model for emotional expression. This closes the door on emotional intimacy for many men.

ISSUES WITH INTIMACY

We all come to relationships with our own set of baggage, but in the area of intimacy, there are three common issues I see with men:

- Inability to sustain a long-term relationship
- Being put in the "friend zone" rather than viewed as boyfriend material
- Being emotionally unavailable

I see lots of single men who have either never been married or are serial monogamists, hopping from one relationship to the next. In true classic avoidant attachment style, these men often had neglectful or emotionally absent mothers, or mothers who were so emotionally dysregulated that they created unstable and erratic attachment patterns. Not surprisingly, there is a high percentage of these men in the dating pool, especially in the San Francisco Bay Area. The world of polyamory and open relationships tends to attract avoidant men and women. The "poly lifestyle" as it is called works well for those with avoidant tendencies. It worked for me the first few years after my divorce. In that community, it's easy and normal to jump from one lover to the next and avoid real emotional intimacy with anyone on a long-term basis.

Men who are afraid of women and who do not know how to step into their masculine power often end up in platonic relationships with women they'd rather be romantic with. Typically, these men had very strong, domineering mothers who did not give them sufficient independence to figure out their own problems. This can emasculate young boys, and as adults, they either look for domineering women who can take care of them or are repeatedly rejected by potential romantic partners who see them as too needy.

Perpetually in the Friend Zone: Victor's Story

Victor, a forty-year-old single man, struggled with romantic relationships with women. He had many female friends, some of whom he was very attracted to, but these friendships never moved into romance. While Victor was tall and handsome, he lacked confidence around women. He didn't know how to approach a woman, engage her in conversation, or initiate any type of touch. He didn't have a dominant bone in his body and constantly allowed women—and men—to walk all over him. Most women saw Victor as weak and needy. They found him charming in his own way but were not romantically attracted to him. The few women with whom he did become romantically involved left him with a broken heart because his neediness and lack of confidence drove them away. Victor had to take a hard look at himself, including some uncomfortable truths about his mother. In time, he was better able to see how his actions were a turnoff to potential partners. As he stepped into his own power, he became much more comfortable with intimacy. He learned key confidence-building skills and began dating again.

Emotional Detachment: Why Crying is So Good for You

A key block to intimacy for both men and women is emotional detachment and the inability to access one's own emotions, especially sadness. This was definitely a huge issue in my life. I could not cry except when I was watching a movie or reading a book. In that context, one step removed, I could feel sadness and grief, but I remained unable to feel those emotions in my own life. I was overwhelmed when emotions bubbled up and felt I had to push them down. My repressed emotions expressed themselves as anxiety and in the panic attacks I experienced in the middle of the night for decades.

My repressed sadness and grief also expressed themselves in the form of anger and incessant quarreling with my husband. I was exhausted from trying to give him constant emotional support and resented feeling as if I had a third child to parent. My role as the cheerleader wife turned into my being the taskmaster, which made him feel even more inadequate and repeated the pattern he'd experienced with his parents. He, too, was unable to fully access his emotions, and this was complicated by deep-seated anger and disappointment. He became explosive at times, with doors slamming and extremely high levels of tension in the air. There was never any physical threat to the kids or me, but he injured himself more than once by punching a wall or kicking a door.

The funny thing about repressed emotions is that eventually they come to the surface, often in unexpected ways. Several years after my separation, I spent the better part of a year grieving my first post-separation relationship with a guy I call "Boston Man."

Far from being an ideal pairing, my relationship with this man was downright abusive at times. My friends hated how he treated me and were thrilled when I broke up with him. But I thought he was the love of my life. I was beyond heartbroken and would walk through New York City sobbing every time I saw a street, restaurant, hotel, or park bench where we had been together. My therapist told me again and again that my grief was not about Boston Man but the loss of my father, for whom I had never been able to grieve. It took years of personal development and growth to realize how right he was.

A common pattern for emotionally detached individuals is getting into relationships with other emotionally detached individuals. This prevents both parties from being vulnerable and ensures that true intimacy will not occur. This was definitely my pattern, both in my marriage and in some of my early post-separation relationships.

Intimacy Requires an Emotional Connection

While emotional detachment has many negative consequences in one's entire life, it is particularly detrimental when it comes to sex and intimacy. For most women, deep passionate sex happens when they have an emotional connection. In that space of connection, trust, and safety, women can fully open themselves up sexually and experience intense sexual pleasure. When intimacy is lacking and a woman does not feel connected or safe, it is extremely difficult for her to surrender fully into her sexuality. The vulnerability required to surrender can best happen when there's a strong emotional connection. This tends not to be the case as much with men, who are more comfortable expressing pleasure. This saying from one of my Tantra teachers sums up the impasse: "A man wants into a woman's Yoni (vagina) and a woman wants into a man's heart."

Most securely attached women have "emotional radar," and they can pretty quickly assess a man's emotional capacity and availability. If a man is unavailable emotionally, they might hang around for a bit to see if they can break through the wall, but if that doesn't happen pretty quickly, they lose interest. This doesn't necessarily preclude good sex, but without emotional intimacy, there is no potential for a long-term healthy relationship.

Learning How to Let Others Care for Her: Lisa's Story

Lisa had everything going for her. She was a thirty-five-year-old successful, beautiful, intelligent CEO of a growing company. She never had a hard time getting dates; in fact, men flocked to her.

She desperately wanted to find her life partner and start a family. But Lisa kept attracting financially unstable men who saw her as their meal ticket. For the most part, the guys she dated were needy, clingy, and emotionally immature. While Lisa's business instincts were sharp, she had no instincts when it came to men and dating. She learned at an early age that in order to feel loved, she had to take care of others. But the minute she became the caretaker in these relationships, she felt anger and resentment, which caused her to lose all interest in sex. In our sessions, Lisa learned to identify and acknowledge her attachment wounds, practice self-compassion and self-care, and allow others to care for her. This opened the door for her to find her life partner.

Dealing with a Broken Heart: Tristan's Story

People with a broken or wounded heart will also experience emotional detachment and fear of intimacy. Men and women who've been through an acrimonious divorce are understandably afraid to open up to another partner. Tristan came to see me after his wife left him for another man. He was heartbroken and completely perplexed by the sudden end of his marriage. He struggled to connect with women he wanted to date. His cock wouldn't cooperate, and he began having erection issues. When Tristan was five, his mother was hospitalized with cancer and died later that year. His father remarried soon after, but Tristan never formed a bond with his new stepmother, who favored her own children. The separation from Tristan's wife triggered his childhood abandonment issues and made him distrust women. He closed off his heart so that he would not be wounded again when the inevitable rejection came. Tristan had to learn how to reconnect with his emotions and allow himself to grieve for the little boy who had been abandoned. He also realized how his anxious attachment style manifested in neediness and mistrust, which drove his wife away from him. Once Tristan was able to heal these old wounds, his sexual energy and erections returned as well. When I last spoke to Tristan, he was in Europe with a woman he had been dating for over a year.

Those of us with anxious attachment styles often have the opposite problem. Rather than feeling emotionally detached, we become overly attached to a partner. We get needy, desperate, and clingy and frequently end up driving potential partners away. Childhood fears of abandonment and lack of self-worth are often the root causes of this behavior. Sometimes this pattern makes us confuse sex with love and intimacy. Sex and love are two different things and we can choose to have one without the other. However, those with abandonment wounds easily confuse the two, fearing abandonment if they don't have sex and then becoming overly emotionally attached once they do.

Confusing Sex with Love: Caryn's Story

Caryn came to see me because she could not maintain a long-term relationship. Every man she ever got close to ended up leaving her in short order. I could see why. Caryn always became obsessed when she started dating someone. She would text him incessantly, question his every move, and ask for a commitment early on in the relationship. She was, in a word, smothering. What emotionally healthy guy wouldn't bolt? Caryn, like many individuals with anxious attachment issues, confused sex with love and intimacy, so every man she had casual sex with became an instant attachment object. She had a knack for finding emotionally and geographically unavailable men, also a common habit among avoidants. As Caryn began to feel more self-worth and learned to respect other's boundaries, she started enjoying casual sex and learned that it did not have to translate into intimacy. This was an important first step toward her finding a healthy intimate relationship.

Shame, sexual abuse, wounding, and intimacy blocks are all reasons that we become sexually disconnected. The more you understand about your own blueprint and the reasons behind some of your challenges, the better equipped you will be to heal them and transform your life. Change starts with self-knowledge and self-awareness. In Part II of this book, we are going to take a deep dive into what a healing journey might look like. I will help you create your own pathway to sexual healing and awakening, pleasure, and life transformation. You will discover the building blocks for living an orgasmic life.

PART TWO

.

Awakening Your

Pleasure

Chapter 8

BEGINNING THE JOURNEY OF SEXUAL HEALING & AWAKENING

Now that you have an understanding of why we become sexually disconnected, it's time to turn our attention to how you can create a fulfilling sex life. Remember, you can't live an orgasmic life if you are not truly connected with your sexuality. Part II of this book will show you a path forward to reclaim your pleasure. What I most want you to know is that you can heal old wounds and transform this vital aspect of who you are. You can learn to express your desires, set boundaries, and ask for what you want from a lover. All you need is skillful support and the willingness to engage in the challenge with courage and an open heart. I also want you to know that your journey is unique; your experience will differ from that of other women. There is no one right way to reconnect with your sexuality and heal sexual wounds. Be cautious about anyone who tells you the contrary or tries to convince you that they have the perfect technique or program. It's really important for you to feel into your body and heart and decide whether a particular program or teacher is right for you.

Sexual awakening and healing take time. Layers and layers of experiences, emotions, and ways in which the body gets triggered need time to unwind. "Compassion, self-love, and patience" is my mantra and the mantra I recommend to all my clients. It took decades for all of this to be imprinted on you, and it may take some time for your experience of your sexuality to begin to transform. But change will happen as long as you are prepared to put aside false beliefs, heal past wounds, and open yourself up to new experiences.

FOUR GUIDING PRINCIPLES TO TRANSFORMING YOUR SEX LIFE

There are a number of guiding principles inherent to the process of transforming your sex life.

- Self-awareness and the courage to address your issues
- Understanding and banishing your sexual shame
- Accepting and loving your body, especially your vagina
- Allowing yourself to fully experience pleasure

Self-Awareness and Courage

Just by reading this book, you are beginning the process of healing. By acknowledging that you have a problem, that everything is not OK, you are opening the door to change. That very first step is often the hardest. I can't begin to tell you how many women shed uncontrollable tears when they finally make that phone call and reach out for help. Even after that first call, some do not follow up and get the help they so desperately want and need. Others take a year or more after an initial conversation to go the next step and schedule a session. This is totally normal given the fact that sexuality is such a potent part of who we are. Opening the door to healing can be scary, so it's important to approach this endeavor with tender loving care.

How you become self-aware and ready to face what's there will also vary from woman to woman. My own path started with a spiritual awakening, which is not that uncommon. I was in my mid-forties when I started attending Unity Church in Manhattan at the suggestion of some of my best friends who were also Jewish. For someone who was brought up in the Jewish tradition, married a Jewish man, and raised her children Jewish, becoming a regular churchgoer was more than a little unexpected. But Unity Church in Manhattan is a very special and unique place. I felt like I was attending a Broadway show every Sunday morning with the most talented performers in the world! The nondenominational congregation was just as racially and economically diverse as the city itself.

Unity gave me a doorway into my spirituality without having to deal with organized religion. As I meditated and prayed, I began to see how dissatisfied I was with my marriage, how lonely I felt, and how far apart my husband and I had grown. I began to see that my life could be different, that I didn't have to settle for what I had, that there was more. Initially, I hoped that my husband would join me and that Unity would bring us closer. But in actuality, my spiritual life increased the divide. Once again, we did not agree and could not share a vital part of life with each other.

Unity espoused the law of attraction and of gratitude and the belief that God or spirit is inside of each of us. All of this really resonated with me. At the end of the year, I participated in an annual Unity tradition and wrote myself a letter as if the present day was one year from now and I was looking back on the events of the year. That simple exercise was a major turning point in my life. It was the first time I admitted to myself that I wanted to end my marriage. This realization forced me to face the issues around my sexuality. It was the beginning of self-awareness, but it would be years before I began to focus on healing in earnest.

Knowing what you want or don't want in your life is fundamental to living an orgasmic life. It's impossible to manifest a life that flows if you don't comprehend the components of your life. The following visioning exercise I learned at Unity will help you to assess what you want your orgasmic life to look like. Don't be frustrated if it seems unattainable! Just go with the images that you notice. Visions can be both literal and also representative of change that you want to manifest.

Exercise: Visioning Letter

What you will need: paper, pen, self-addressed stamped envelope
Find a quiet place where you can be alone for ten to fifteen minutes. Close your eyes and feel your body on the chair and your feet on the floor. Take a few deep breaths. Identify three to five important parts of your life (e.g., personal relationships, health, career, your interests and passions). Focus on the areas you would like to change. Now envision how your life could be different a year from now. Get as specific as possible. Rather than saying, "A year from now I want to have a great sex life," say, "A year from now I want to feel attractive and sexy, to know that men desire me." Do this visioning for each part of your life you would like to change.

Now write yourself a letter by hand as if it's the present day one year from now. In this letter, talk about what this past year has been like for you. Focus on the changes that have occurred and the impact those changes have had on you and your loved ones. This is a great opportunity to also envision the future for the people who are most important in your life—your partner, children, family members, friends, and colleagues. As you begin writing, other visions may show up. Go with the flow. Don't overthink it. Set a time limit and don't edit the letter. Stream of consciousness writing is very powerful and often helps us connect with hidden parts of our consciousness.

Address the letter to yourself, and then give it to a trusted friend or family member and ask them to mail it to you in a year. Put a tickler in your calendar so you can give them a gentle reminder if you haven't received it.

As my spirituality began to awaken, I noticed a stirring inside of me. It was subtle at first, a deep dissatisfaction and a longing—for what, I did not know. As it became more and more clear that my marriage was over, the stirring became stronger. I found myself starting to notice other men and was shocked when they noticed me back. Shocked because, objectively speaking, I've always been an attractive woman, but I had NEVER felt sexy or attractive. In fact, I went out of my way—all over New York City—to find the most stylish baggy clothes available. That's how uncomfortable it was for me to inhabit my body. It didn't help that my husband rarely complimented my looks and had not told me I was sexy in decades. When you don't get that type of positive reinforcement, you begin to believe that you're not attractive. To this day, I still have a hard time hearing from a man that they think I'm attractive. Yet the more I hear it, the more I begin to believe it. When I work with men, I always emphasize the importance of telling their partner she's hot and sexy and turns him on.

As men began noticing me, I grew more courageous and started flirting. It was a perfect setup: as a part-time Broadway producer, I was always wining and dining potential investors who for the most part were men. I had plenty of opportunity to practice flirting, and as it turned out, I was pretty good at it! Then one day, I had an intrusive thought: "No way I can leave my marriage. I am too broken…what man would want a woman who can't have sex with him?" I mean, can you imagine my OK Cupid dating profile? "Awesome woman, smart, interesting, fun to be with, but she'll never have sex with you." That was not going to fly.

Understanding and Banishing Sexual Shame

The next turning point in my journey was facing my shame. Again, this came about through Unity Church, where I found the courage to face this challenge. It happened at a week-long summer retreat. Little did I know it would be the first of many spiritual retreats that I would attend. We were working on identifying seminal events in our lives. For the first time, I really looked at the incident that had happened when I was nine with my pet dog. This opened up a deep wound, and I found myself journaling furiously about other shameful sexual experiences, the memories of which started coming back to me. While I was not able to share this story until several years later, that particular retreat marked a turning point. A key theme throughout the week was: you are not your story or your past, and you can transform your life. This gave me the fortitude to move forward and leave my husband, knowing that I would somehow come to terms with my sexuality.

My husband and I ended our marriage quite amicably. Once we separated, I began to blossom in ways that I could never have imagined. I shed my baggy clothes and jumped into online dating with gusto. On the few occasions I was intimate with a man, sex continued to be uncomfortable rather than pleasurable. At that point, I began to look for help. When I told my OB/GYN that sex was always painful, she referred me to a pelvic floor physical therapist who diagnosed me with a tight pelvic floor. Treatment involved internal pelvic work, which was extremely uncomfortable and did not address the emotional issues related to painful sex. In addition, I was instructed to use dilators (hard plastic dildos that gradually increase in diameter) so my vagina could get used to penetration again. My vagina did not respond well to this treatment and sex continued to be painful.

Several months after I left my marriage, I started the relationship with Boston Man. He was everything my husband wasn't; tall, confident, and super sexy with piercing blue eyes. It was an odd relationship in that we never had intercourse because he had a girlfriend back in Boston and didn't want to cheat on her. We spent a lot of time together during the week, having dinner and drinks in restaurants around the city and passionately making out in public. There were a few sleepovers and a little bit of light foreplay. Strangers noticed us when we walked down the street arm in arm; the sexual charge between us was that potent. Boston Man loved sexual banter, and I would receive frequent teasing phone calls and texts.

Boston Man also had a dominant side, a novel experience for me and a huge turn-on. I learned a lot about myself from this relationship, although most of it was quite painful. I was devastated when he suddenly left New York and went back to Boston. But I had enough self-awareness to know I was clueless as to how to have a healthy intimate relationship with a man.

For the first time, I was able to see my attachment wounds play out in a relationship. I was petrified of being abandoned, so I did anything to keep him in my life, including allowing myself to continuously be disappointed, rejected, emotionally abused, and mistreated. The best thing that Boston Man did for me was to awaken my desire. I wanted to have sex with him more than anything, and by denying me that, he ignited and fanned the flame. I literally came home from our dates dripping wet and could not wait to get out my vibrator. Today, if I see a client enacting this type of pattern where teasing leads to a massive turn-on that cannot be consummated, I talk with them about the dynamic. This kind of teasing followed by being denied sex can easily turn sexual attraction into an addiction. With the sexual attention comes a rush of dopamine (the "feel good" hormone) that keeps us coming back for more, hoping that this time will be different and we'll get what we crave. But we never do, and the cycle continues to our detriment until such time as the relationship changes or ends.

Accepting and Loving Your Body

This third guiding principle, body love and acceptance, is one of the most challenging, especially for women. It took me several years to learn to love my body, especially my pussy. To be honest, I still struggle with this at times. A major breakthrough happened when I attended a women's retreat. In the healing circle, women talked about their relationship with their body, especially their Yoni, womb, and other sex organs. The stories were so powerful and so relatable. Here were all these women who like me had suffered shame and embarrassment about their periods. Many women talked about sexual abuse. When one woman shared her story about giving birth to her daughter, and how traumatic her labor had been, it all clicked for me. Suddenly I saw how I'd become disconnected from my vagina. Body shaking, voice quivering I stood up in that circle and shared my story. It shocked me when I heard myself talking about miserable pregnancies, constant infections, and the pain I had suffered at the hands of urologists. At that moment, I realized that the physical trauma from twenty-five years ago still lived in my body. Then the "aha" moment came. My vagina closed up during sex because she was protecting me, not punishing me. She did not want me to feel pain. For the first time in my life, I felt compassion rather than repulsion for my vagina.

Exercise: Create Your Vagina Timeline

In this exercise from Tami Lynn Kent's book, *Wild Feminine*, you are going to create a vagina timeline that will help you recognize experiences that have shaped you as a woman. This exercise helps us identify major events in our life specifically related to our female body, sexuality, and femininity.

1. Draw a line lengthwise across a piece of paper to represent your timeline from conception to present. Divide your age in half and write this number at the center point of your timeline. Divide each half of the timeline into sections, each representing a decade of your life.

2. Identify events associated with your female body or sense of your femininity that impacted you in some way. Listen to your intuition and write down whatever comes to you. Sometimes those seemingly minor events end up being very important.

3. Spend some time considering what's on the timeline and ponder these questions:

   - Would you characterize your initial relationship with your female body as positive or negative?
   - How did that relationship change over time?
   - What were the seminal events that caused a change in your relationship with your female body?
   - How did the relationship with your female body impact your sexuality and feminine nature?

What did you learn from this exercise? Were there events that you wrote about that surprised you? Let's hear for a moment about some other women's experiences with their vagina timeline.

My Period Betrayed Me: Bethany's Story

"I was fourteen years old, and my mom had finally relented and let me shop downtown all by myself. I felt an immense amount of freedom and relished the opportunity to be treated like an adult by the shopkeepers. The day was hot and sticky, and as I walked along the street, I felt prickles of sweat starting to fall down my back. New sneakers in the window of the shoe store caught my attention, so I went in to try them on. Mr. Clark, who had waited on me since I was a kid and knew my entire family, was standing behind the counter with a friendly smile on his face. As I walked up to the counter, I noticed that I was feeling wet around my thighs. I looked down and to my horror saw blood on my white shorts. My period had come, and I didn't have any pads with me. Mr. Clark noticed too and quickly ushered me into the bathroom, where I made a makeshift pad with toilet paper. Luckily, I had a jacket and wrapped it around my waist. I used his phone and called my mom to pick me up. I was so mortified that after this incident I refused to go into the store when Mr. Clark was there. To this day, every time I pass that store I get a sick feeling in my stomach. This incident made me hate my period and my body because I felt like it had totally betrayed me."

Where Did My Beautiful Body Go?: Julia's Story

"I always loved my body. I had great boobs, a really tight stomach from all my exercising, and not a bit of cellulite in my thighs. I proudly wore my bikinis and loved showing off my 'stuff' on the beach. Mike told me that he first fell in love with me when he saw me running around in my bikini playing Frisbee with my dog. Two babies later and I can't even look at myself in the mirror. My boobs sag and are all swollen from breastfeeding. I will never wear a bikini again because of the awful stretchmarks on my belly. My belly will not flatten even with me doing two hundred sit ups a day. My thighs jiggle when I walk. We have sex under the sheets because I am too embarrassed for Mike to really see me. I seriously want to take this body and trade it in for another one."

Menopause Madness: Laina's Story

"Menopause hit me like a ton of bricks. One day I was a totally normal forty-eight-year-old woman and the next day I was a raving lunatic. I couldn't sleep at night because of the night sweats. It was thirty degrees in the city and I walked around without a coat. Brain fog overtook me, and I couldn't remember where I put my keys, what I was supposed to be doing next, or the password to my bank account. I cried at the drop of a hat, raged at the gas station attendant because the pump wasn't working, and felt perpetually tired and cranky. I had no desire to have sex. In fact, the thought of it repulsed me. My body had a mind of its own and I was just along for the ride."

There are so many ways in which women feel betrayed by our bodies throughout our lives. Distancing yourself from your body makes the journey of coming back to it even harder. Next time you feel angry with your body, see if you can turn that anger into compassion and acceptance. Getting on the same page as your body is the first step toward coming home to your body and finding your pleasure.

Embodiment—The Place to Begin

Your sexual healing journey begins somatically, as you connect with your body. Embodiment is an experiential awareness of the feelings and sensations within our body or the reality that we "live in our skin." Unfortunately, many abuse and trauma survivors do not feel safe being in their body. It can also take some time to reconnect with your body if you've been disconnected for a long period.

I start out all my clients with embodiment practices. You must be connected to your own body before you can truly connect with a partner. Grounding is the first step toward embodiment so that you can be completely present and in the moment. The next step is to notice sensations in the body. Embodiment practices are best taught using audio so that you can close your eyes and focus on sensations. If you'd like to learn a series of embodiment practices, head over to this website and sign up for a free fourteen-day Body Awakening Adventure: www.myawakebody.com.

In the next chapter, you will learn in detail about one woman's personal journey to finding pleasure and orgasmic bliss.

Chapter 9

COMING HOME TO MY BODY AND WELCOMING PLEASURE

Welcoming Pleasure

Finding pleasure in my body came to me slowly. Boston Man stoked the flames, but it was Tantra Man, Eric, who became my sexual healer, starting with the beautiful night of Goddess worship. Eric had initially studied Tantra with Charles Muir, who emphasizes the sexual healing aspects of Tantra. With his gentle touch, great skill, and technique, as well as his amazing patience and desire to support my awakening, my body began responding as layers of shame began to melt. There were times when I was sufficiently relaxed and aroused to have pain-free, pleasurable intercourse, which was a first for me. I began to experience pleasure when he massaged my G-spot, although that type of orgasm was still elusive because I could not fully surrender.

Eric also taught me how to run sexual energy in my body, a completely new concept to me. Running sexual energy involves using breath to create a circuitous path of energy that runs from the genitals to the top of the head. He was very connected to his own energy, so we had many juicy sessions of exchanging energy through breath. My experience of sex began to change as I saw how Tantra could help me bond with a partner in a completely different way, bringing more sensation and connection into the relationship.

When Eric told me that Charles Muir, who was based on the West Coast, was teaching a workshop in Boston, I jumped at the chance to experience his work and at the opportunity to reconnect with Boston Man. The workshop was a huge success, but staying with Boston Man was a disaster. He predictably snuck out in the middle of the night and went to his home in Nantucket, as well as to see a new girlfriend he'd failed to tell me about.

I was extremely challenged by the eye gazing exercise in Charles Muir's workshop. Maintaining any type of eye contact was difficult, and I had this horrible habit of closing my eyes when I spoke to someone. A number of people accused me of being rude or dismissive. The truth was that looking into someone's eyes was way too vulnerable for me. The exercise had us maintaining eye contact with a partner while answering the question: "What are you afraid of?" Much to my surprise, I answered, "Losing myself sexually."

Later that evening, I paired up with a complete stranger, who had been instructed in the workshop how to perform sacred spot (G-spot) massage and how to hold space for a woman during a sexual healing session by being totally present with her. Again, I was surprised that I allowed myself to completely let go and experience pleasure. Miraculously, nothing bad happened to me. No longer a complete stranger, my partner was totally supportive and encouraged me to express myself—to scream, cry, and make loud, unladylike noises. I felt huge waves of relief and ecstasy wash over my body as I allowed myself to finally accept and celebrate that I am a sexual being who deserves to experience enormous pleasure. I was now on my way to sexual awakening and healing.

The Road to Becoming a Sex and Intimacy Coach

Over the next several years, I continued my healing journey, and it goes on to this day. I experienced the power of hands-on work and eventually moved to California where all of the programs and teachers from whom I wanted to learn were based. In fairly rapid succession, I signed up for every sexuality and Tantra program I could find the time to participate in. Within a year of my having moved to the West Coast, I left my job to pursue a career in sexual awakening and healing even though I still had no idea what that would look like or how it would pay the bills. My mom's death from Alzheimer's disease at the age of ninety-four provided me with a huge gift. She left me some money, which allowed me to take a year off and focus entirely on training for my new profession.

I went about this the only way a person trained as a lawyer knew—as if I were literally getting a doctoral degree. Over the next year and a half, I took four different intensive training programs. I started with Charles Muir's Source School of Tantra teacher training and became certified in his form of Tantra, which focuses on sexual healing. I received numerous hands-on healing sessions from my fellow students, men who helped me release more shame and open up sexually. It was also during this program that I learned how to ejaculate, which was a major goal of the program. Source Tantra prepared me to be a Dakini. Derived from Sanskrit, a Dakini is a Tantric Priestess of ancient India and a practitioner of Tantric Yoga. The word has been appropriated to mean a female sexual healer who works with men providing sensual massage and erotic touch. However, I was pretty certain this was not my path, though I tried it for a few months. I understand the value of the work and the powerful healing it offers men, but maintaining boundaries was exhausting. Also, I was pretty sure it would not pass my litmus test: feeling comfortable with telling my sons what I was doing for a living.

Sexological Bodywork

Next, I was certified as a Sexological Bodyworker through the Institute of the Advanced Study of Human Sexuality. This edgy program played a huge role in my sexual healing. Sexological Bodywork is a somatic (body-based) hands-on sex education modality that helps clients embody their erotic nature through one-way touch. Unlike some sensual massage, Sexological Bodywork is not interactive and abides by a professional code of ethics that requires the practitioner to be fully dressed and use latex gloves for genital touch. The profession is legal in the State of California, which meant it passed my litmus test and assuaged my other concerns.

The Sexological Bodywork training has a didactic component that includes the detailed study of sexual anatomy, the role of the sympathetic and parasympathetic nervous system in sexual arousal, extensive touch skills and techniques, breathing practices, and business development and marketing. My analytical side loved the didactic component, as did my entrepreneurial and creative sides, which began actively figuring out how to create a legitimate business.

The education I received in Sexological Bodywork was also crucial to my personal growth and development. For the first time, I had the opportunity to work with women and touch a lot of different vulvas. That was mind-blowing for me because I saw firsthand how each woman's vulva was unique and how each had a completely different arousal pattern.

One session with a female student will always stand out for me. It was only my second or third time working with a woman. And let me tell you, it is nerve-wracking not knowing what you are going to encounter when you start touching a woman's genitals! Sometimes just finding the clitoris is an adventure in itself. I was filled with anxiety before we even started the session, because like many students in the class, she was much more experienced sexually than I and even did sensual massage for a living. Moreover, I was being observed by another classmate and feared both participants would judge me as inadequate.

After doing my best to give my practice partner a relaxing sensual massage, I finally got the courage to look at her vulva. To my surprise, she had a really large hood covering her clitoris. I was clueless. Even when I lifted it up, which was challenging in itself, I wasn't sure exactly where her clitoris was. She did not enjoy my touch and asked me to stop, as I was triggering a trauma reaction. That session was definitely not one of my shining moments, but I learned a lot from the experience.

I have so much empathy for men because they never know what they are going to find from woman to woman: big hood, small hood, no hood, clitoris that moves around during stimulation, different shaped labia, or vaginal openings that are hard to find. The list goes on and on.

Women's vaginas are fascinating and beautiful. There has been a renewed appreciation for the beauty and variety of women's vaginas in the past few years.

Here are some resources to check some out yourself:

- *Femalia*, a picture book by Joani Blank
- http://www.greatwallofvagina.co.uk/home
- http://www.vulvalovelovely.com/pages/about-us/ (Vulva art)
- https://www.youtube.com/watch?v=Dp8-dYvEfuk (Women's reactions to pictures of their vaginas versus their partners' reactions).

The Sexological Bodywork program cut through a whole other layer of my sexual shame by pushing one of my biggest edges—giving and receiving erotic embodiment sessions in a group of people. In this setting, where pleasure and orgasms were celebrated, I was able to let go and surrender. Feeling erotic and orgasmic energy run through the entire room was exhilarating and brought me to higher levels of sexual expression. However, Sexological Bodywork's somewhat exclusive focus on pleasure did not deal sufficiently with healing sexual wounds and trauma, which made me realize that I needed to have additional tools before I could hang out my shingle.

SkyDancing Tantra
Teacher Training

I had taken a SkyDancing Tantra workshop earlier in the year and really enjoyed the practices and rituals I had learned, which were very different than what was taught at Source School of Tantra. I immediately realized that this was the Tantra lineage with which I wanted to become involved. The day after I completed Sexological Bodywork training in San Francisco, I went to Harbin Hot Springs to begin a seven-month SkyDancing Tantra Teacher training program with Steve and Lokita Carter's Ecstatic Living Institute. I was a woman on a mission.

Many of the SkyDancing Tantra practices have become an integral part of my sex coaching, even though my non-woo-woo clients don't know we're actually doing Tantra. SkyDancing was my first in-depth study of Tantra, as well as the program in which I learned how to be a teacher and to facilitate groups. To my delight, I was good at both, and I am proud to be a member of the Institute's faculty.

Somatica: The Glue that Holds it All Together

During my Sexological Bodywork training, we were visited by Celeste Hirschman and Danielle Harel, former program leaders. They talked about their upcoming new sex and intimacy coaching program based on The Somatica® Method, a body-based approach to sexuality designed to help clients connect with their erotic energy and learn intimacy skills, all without taking their clothes off. This definitely piqued my interest, but when we did an exercise of connecting erotically with another person, I completely freaked out. I felt totally exposed and incredibly uncomfortable. It was one thing to help a client experience pleasure on a massage table, but quite another to bring my own still highly repressed sexuality into the equation. I was absolutely certain I was never going to take their program.

Fast-forward six months, and I find myself sitting in Celeste's living room in Module Two of the Somatica Core Training Program. One of my good friends, who is now my co-teacher, had persuaded me to enroll despite having missed the first weekend and Module One. She said it would rock my world, and truer words had never been spoken.

The Somatica Method is an experiential body-based approach to help clients express and expand their sexuality, learn how to create intimacy, and heal emotional and sexual wounds. For me, it is the glue that holds all of the many tools in my tool belt together. It is the foundation of my coaching work and educational programs. It combines elements of Tantra (eye contact, breath, movement, moving sexual energy), elements of Somatic Experiencing and trauma work, interactive exercises, and adult attachment theory, woven into one comprehensive, extraordinarily powerful curriculum. Since I am also a Sexological Bodyworker, I also incorporate hands-on bodywork for certain clients (e.g., orgasm coaching for women and helping men learn how to control early ejaculation).

After all this training, I finally understood the difference between women's sexuality and men's sexuality and how to work with each. For example, the difference in the arousal pattern of women versus men is often one of the major problems for couples. Men literally wear their arousal equipment on the outside of their body, and it does not take much for a man to get aroused. Men are also quite visual, so looking at a hot woman, let alone having his cock touched, can easily arouse a man. Because of this, men are much more connected to their sexuality and desire for sex. A man's desire often comes before arousal. Women, on the other hand, wear all of their arousal equipment inside their body with the exception of breasts and nipples, but even these tend to be very sensitive if a woman is not yet aroused. Women get aroused from the outside in and take much longer to become sufficiently aroused to be ready for sex.

Unlike with men, a woman's desire for sex usually follows arousal. The more aroused a woman is, the more she wants sex. For women, orgasm begets orgasm. Most men don't understand this and assume that women's arousal is similar to theirs. Touch her pussy and she's ready. Definitely not true. This is one of the most common problems in relationships. The woman is not aroused enough, so when they do have sex, it doesn't feel great to her. Bad sex keeps a woman's libido low. She'd rather do something with her time that is less work and more rewarding than having bad sex.

From my own sexual healing perspective, my Somatica training and coaching have significantly changed the way I view and enter relationships. I learned so much about my own attachment wounds. I struggled with allowing myself to be vulnerable and feel those emotions, which finally began to melt that hard New York lawyer exterior. What emerged from underneath was a caring, compassionate coach and healer who guides and facilitates others to heal sexual wounds, overcome intimacy blocks, and navigate the many challenges of relationship. I did not know at the time that I was also on the way to living an orgasmic life.

Chapter 10

SO WHAT IS TANTRA ANYWAY?

As you already know, Tantra has played a very important part in my sexual healing and awakening. Regardless of whether or not Tantra is in your future, understanding the principles of Tantra will help you in your own sexual journey. I use these principles and many Tantra practices all the time in my coaching practice, even when I am not officially teaching Tantra to my clients.

When you hear the word "Tantra," what's the first image that comes to your mind? If you're like most people, you likely conjure up an image of a man and woman embracing in a sitting position known as yab-yum. You might even imagine multiple people making love at an orgy. These are the most common responses to this question; however, they are a complete misconception of what Tantra really is—a spiritual practice that began in India more than 3,000 years ago. Tantra is a Sanskrit word derived from the root *tan*, which means "to expand." While each school of Tantra has a different interpretation of its meaning, the one that resonates with me is "to weave." In Margot Anand's book, *The Art of Everyday Ecstasy* , she defines Tantra as "the art of weaving the often-contradictory aspects of our self or personality into a unified whole for the purpose of expanding our consciousness."[9]

---

9 Margot Anand, *The Art of Everyday Ecstasy: The Seven Tantric Keys for Bringing Passion, Spirit and Joy into Every Part of Your Life* (Broadway Books, 1998).

Origins of Tantra

When Tantra began in India circa 600–800 AD, Hinduism and Buddhism were the popular religions. A core belief of both of these was that achieving enlightenment, a state of total awakening and bliss often referred to as "nirvana," involved giving up worldly pleasures. Common practices included meditation, yogic postures, fasting, and chanting mantras. Tantra also promised enlightenment, but unlike Hinduism and Buddhism, Tantra embraced worldly pleasures. Tantra practitioners (Tantrikas) cultivated ecstasy and bliss as the means to achieve enlightenment. Yoga postures, meditation, and mantras were all part of Tantra. But unlike their Buddhist counterparts who were living ascetic lives, Tantrikas feasted on good food and wine. They sang, danced, and celebrated all parts of life, including sexuality. According to Andre Padoux's *The Roots of Tantra*:

> Tantra provides a synthesis between spirit and matter to enable man to achieve his fullest spiritual and material potential. Renunciation, detachment, and asceticism—by which one may free oneself from the bondage of existence and thereby recall one's original identity with the source of the universe—are not the way of Tantra... Tantra is the opposite: not a withdrawal from life, but the fullest possible acceptance of our desires, feelings, and situations as human beings.[10]

To be clear, Tantra does not advocate adopting a hedonistic life style. One must make conscious choices and choose with discrimination which actions will lead one toward awakening and spiritual bliss.

---

10 André Padoux, *The Roots of Tantra*. State University of New York Press, 2001.

Hinduism and Buddhism were patriarchal systems; women were denigrated and made subordinate to men. Tantra was quite different. In Tantra, not only were men and women treated equally, women were venerated and even worshipped. In Tantric mythology, the great God Shiva, god of pure consciousness, was united with the Goddess Shakti, the goddess of pure energy. Like Shiva, Shakti was powerful—a yogini who embodied pure energy. The source of her power came from her Yoni (vagina), her secret garden; she was the mother of all creation. When her Yoni and his Lingam (penis) came together in sacred union, Shiva and Shakti took their place as the mother and father of the world.

This is a sex-positive, alternative view of the Adam and Eve story. Shakti and Shiva were worshipped in ancient times. When I visited Thailand, Vietnam, and Cambodia a few years ago, I saw many ancient ruins and temples. Every single one had Yoni and Lingam statues. In the temples at Angkor Wat in Cambodia, the largest religious monument in the world created in the twelfth century, there are murals depicting the union of Shiva and Shakti and many Lingam and Yoni statues.

Tantra also provided paths that were focused more on meditation and yoga and put less emphasis on the sexual component. Regardless of the path you chose, the ultimate goal of Tantra was to achieve enlightenment and bliss. One of the key ways to achieve enlightenment was by using sexual energy to accelerate spiritual development. The Tantrikas realized the potency of sexual energy to transform consciousness through holding back orgasmic release. Men were trained, and still are, to have non-ejaculatory sex and use their arousal to connect with a higher level of consciousness.

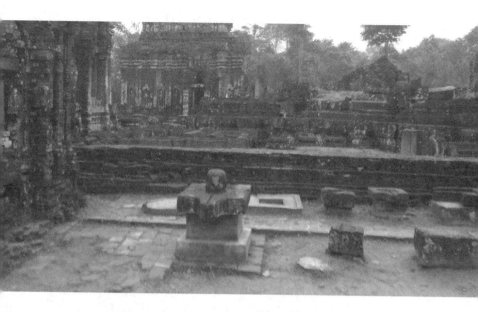

Yoni Statute, My Son Temple Ruins, Vietnam, 14th Century

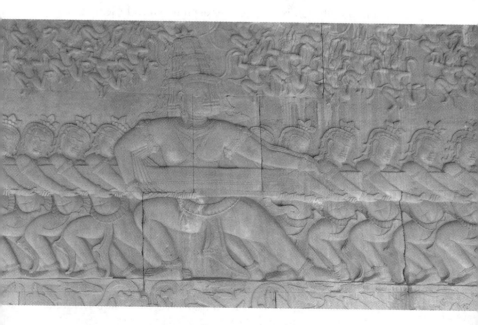

Mural representation of Shiva battle, Angkor Wat, Cambodia,
12th century

The Emergence of
SkyDancing Tantra

Tantra came to the western world in the 1960s and 1970s during the era of free love; it is often referred to as "Neo-Tantra." The Indian guru Bhagwan Shree Rajneesh, who later changed his name to Osho, was largely responsible for bringing Tantra to the west. Osho embraced sexual activity with a partner or partners as a means to achieving bliss. He espoused sexual love as an art and as a skillful sexual practice. According to Osho, "Tantra is the science of transforming ordinary lovers into soul mates. And that is the grandeur of Tantra. It can transform the whole earth." Margot Anand, in her bestselling book, *The Art of Sexual Ecstasy* further elucidates, "[Tantra] acknowledges that sex is at the root of life and that to make human sexuality and erotic union a form of worship and meditation is to practice reverence for life, leading us directly through the pleasure of the senses to spiritual liberation."[11]

Margot Anand met Osho in his ashram in India and became one of his early disciples, tasked with leading Tantra workshops at his ashram. Years of Tantric practice and ritual, as well as her work as a psychotherapist and bodyworker, culminated in the development of SkyDancing Tantra. Often called the "Grandmother of Western Tantra," one of Anand's greatest contributions was to codify the philosophy and practices of Western Tantra, since like other eastern religious practices, Tantra had previously only been taught as an oral tradition. Anand wrote three seminal books, *The Art of Sexual Ecstasy*, *The Art of Everyday Ecstasy*, and *The Art of Sexual Magic*, and gave birth to SkyDancing Tantra Institute Worldwide. I had the great fortune to train with Steve and Lokita

11 Margot Anand, *The Art of Sexual Ecstasy: The Path of Sacred Sexuality for Western Lovers* (Tarcher/Putnam, 1989).

Carter, at the time Margot Anand's lineage holders in the US, who had founded and directed the official SkyDancing Tantra Institute USA, the Ecstatic Living Institute.

In SkyDancing Tantra, I learned a much softer, gentler, and more spiritual approach to Tantra that deeply resonated with me. Unlike Charles Muir's philosophy, which utilized Tantric practices solely for the purpose of sexual healing, SkyDancing Tantra helped me learn how to use my sexual energy with or without a partner to connect with higher consciousness. Said simply, SkyDancing Tantra brings spirit into the bedroom.

> This is the Tantric definition of our sexuality: the return to absolute innocence, absolute oneness. The greatest sexual thrill of all is not a search for thrills, but a silent waiting— utterly relaxed, utterly mindless. One is conscious, conscious only of being conscious. One is consciousness.
>
> —Osho

Some of the practices Margot Anand incorporated into SkyDancing Tantra are aimed at sexual healing, but they take a much gentler approach than those taught by Charles Muir. I will never forget the first time I did the "Yoni Talk" exercise where we learned how to listen to our Yoni. Mine was quite vocal and had lots of good information to pass on. Let's find out what messages your Yoni wants to impart to you.

Exercise: The Yoni Talk

From "The Love & Ecstasy Training (LET)®" shared with special permission by Margot Anand:

Find twenty minutes of uninterrupted time. Create a special space. Light some candles, put on some music, and dress in a sarong or lingerie (anything out of the ordinary). Lie down on your back, close your eyes, and place your right hand over your heart chakra (right in the middle of your chest) and your left hand over your Yoni. Spend three to five minutes breathing deeply into your pelvis so that you feel the hand on your Yoni rise and fall. Begin to visualize a rose or lotus flower and notice how the petals start to gently open as you continue to breathe. Without having any goals or expectations, ask your Yoni some questions and see what she has to say.

- How are you feeling today?
- How am I treating you?
- What do you need?
- What could I do differently?
- What advice do you have for me?

If you are struggling with a particular issue, this is a great time to ask your Yoni for her advice on how to handle it. Don't be surprised if this gets emotional. If you start crying or getting angry, just allow yourself to be with your emotions and stay with them until they pass. You can also check in and see if your Yoni has a name. Often this will show up as some sort of visualization. My Yoni's name is Lilac. When your Yoni is finished talking to you, write down everything that you heard or learned. You will want to look back at it frequently. If this exercise feels challenging, don't despair. It often takes a few attempts before you can begin to really connect with your Yoni.

Chakras and Sexual Awakening

SkyDancing Tantra gave me a new appreciation for the importance of chakras in sexual awakening and healing. According to Anodea Judith, author of *The Chakra System*, this energy center map, which comes from the Tantric tradition, focuses on the subtle body, the nonphysical body that is superimposed on our physical bodies. It can be measured as electromagnetic force fields within and around all living creatures."[12]

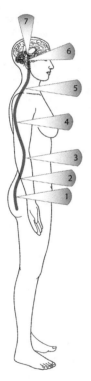

7th Chakra—Pituitary Gland

6th Chakra—Pineal Gland

5th Chakra—Thyroid Gland

4th Chakra—Thymus Gland

3rd Chakra—Pancreas

2nd Chakra—Ovaries and Testes

1st Chakra—Adrenal Glands

The body contains seven chakras that are located along the spinal column near the seven major spinal nerve centers in the body. These energy centers start from the sacrum/perineum area and go all the way to the top of the head.

You can envision them as positioned within an inner flute or hollow tube that runs vertically in front of the spine. Judith describes these energy centers as wheels that spin in a circular fashion. They are often depicted as lotus flowers with a different number of petals

---

12 Anodea Judith, *Wheels of Life: A Journey Through the Chakras.* © 1999 Llewellyn Worldwide, Ltd., 1999. 2143 Wooddale Drive, Woodbury, MN 55125. All rights reserved, used with permission.

for each chakra. Like a flower, they "can be open or closed, dying or budding, depending on the state of consciousness within." Per Judith, "The chakras are gateways between various dimensions—centers where the activity of one dimension, such as emotion and thought, connects and plays on another dimension, such as our physical bodies." Connecting with the chakras, which is the key to circulating sexual energy, helps one to feel the flow of energy within your body. This flow is another building block for accessing orgasmic life energy.

Exercise: Subtle Energy

In this exercise you will have an opportunity to experience your subtle energy body.

Close your eyes and rub your hands together for ten seconds or until you feel a lot of heat generated in your hands. Now move your hands apart six inches so they are still facing each other. Focus your attention on the center of your palms in each hand. Visualize that you are holding a small ball between your hands. Now slowly start to move your hands together and notice any sensation that you are feeling between your two hands. Then slowly start to move your hands apart. Again, notice any sensation. You might even feel some resistance. When you feel some sensation, you are experiencing your energy field. If you don't feel anything, continue to try this. Sometimes it takes a bit of practice to start to feel the sensation.

Chakras can be open and flowing or closed and blocked. They also can be excessive or deficient. For example, a person who is very greedy will often have an overactive first chakra, because they are constantly struggling for survival and abundance. Someone with a deficient third chakra, the power center, may be meek and allow themselves to constantly be taken advantage of. The state of your chakras can vary widely and can also be changed by certain situations.

Each of the chakras is connected to an emotional as well as a physical component. In the chakra chart below, you can see that each chakra also has a color and an earth element. These energy centers have always shown up in our vernacular. For example, your third chakra, which is in your belly, is your power center; that is where the saying "fire in the belly" derives from. But when the third chakra is blocked, anxiety and fear show up—hence, "butterflies in your stomach." Similarly, the fifth chakra, located in the throat, is about being able to speak your truth. But when you can't, you may have a "frog in your throat."

CHAKRA COLORS & MEANINGS

CROWN
Sahasara
Violet
Top of the Head
Thought

▶ **Enlightenment & Spirituality Consciousness**
Excessive: Overly Intellectual, Confusion,
Spiritual Addiction, Dissociation
Deficient: Limited Beliefs, Apathy
Balanced: Wisdom, Knowledge, Spiritual
Connection, Consciousness

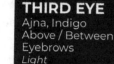

THIRD EYE
Ajna, Indigo
Above / Between
Eyebrows
Light

▶ **Intuition & Understanding**
Excessive: Headaches, Nighmares, Delusions,
Difficulty, Concentrating
Deficient: Poor Memory, Poor Vision,
Unimaginitive, Dental
Balanced: Psychic Perception, Accurate
Interpretation, Imagination, Clear Seeing

THROAT
Vishuddha
Blue
Center base of Neck
Sound

▶ **Comminucation & Self - Expression**
Excessive: Inability to Listen, Stuttering
Excessive Talking
Deficient: Fear of Speaking, Poor Rythm
Balanced: Clear Communication, Creativity, Resonance

HEART
Anahata
Green
Center of Chest
Air

▶ **Balance, Love & Connection**
Excessive: Codependency, Jealous, Possessive,
Poor Boundaries
Deficient: Shy, Lonely, Isolated, Bitter
Balanced: Compassion, Balance, Self Acceptance,
Good Relationships

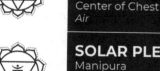

SOLAR PLEXUS
Manipura
Yellow
Below Sternum
Fire

▶ **Energy, Vitality, Will Power, Desire,
Personal Authority**
Excessive: Dominating, Controlling, Aggressive,
Scattered
Deficient: Poor Self Esteem, Passive
Balanced: Vitality, Strength of Will, Purpose, Self Esteem

SACRAL
Svadhisthana
Orange
Below Navel
Water

▶ **Relationship, Emotions & Sexuality,
Self Gratification**
Excessive: Overly Emotional, Sex Addiction,
Obsessive Attachments
Deficient: Rigid, Emotionally Numb
Balanced: Healthy Sexually, Pleasure, Feeling, Fluidity

ROOT
Muladhara
Red
Base of Spine
Earth

▶ **To Be Here, Grounded, Survival,
Self Preservation**
Excessive: Obesity, Greed, Materialism,
Hoarding, Sluggish
Deficient: Fearful, Underweight, Spacey
Balanced: Stability, Grounded, Prosperity,
Physically Healthy, Trust

While all of the seven chakras are equally important and work together as a whole integrated system, the lower chakras are most relevant to your sexuality. Your first chakra, also called the **Root chakra**, is located in the sacrum/perineum area. This chakra is about survival and feeling grounded, secure, and safe. There is also a sexual aspect to your Root chakra, which can be accessed through the anus, a primary pleasure center. If you experienced economic or physical hardships growing up, if your physical safety was threatened in any way, or if you have been in emotionally unstable relationships, you will likely have some blockages in the first chakra.

The second chakra, called the **Sacral chakra**, is located below your belly button and encompasses all of your sex organs. This chakra is the center of sexuality and creativity. A woman's vagina is the nexus of her creative power; when this chakra is open, your sexuality and creativity will flow. Orgasmic life force energy comes from this chakra. When it's open and flowing, you have the ability to create new life, not just human life, but new businesses, new relationships, new opportunities, and new ideas. This is central to the process of living an orgasmic life. Unfortunately, the second chakra can easily become blocked, especially if you've experienced sexual abuse, sexual trauma, or physical wounding, including childbirth. If this chakra is blocked, you might lose your libido, feel numb, have a hard time experiencing sensations and pleasure, or have challenges with orgasm. It is for this reason that we must first address our sexual wounds if we wish to live an orgasmic life.

The third chakra, called the **Solar Plexus chakra**, is located between your solar plexus and your belly button and occupies most of the belly. This chakra is where personal power and will resides. It is the "fire in the belly" chakra. When it is open, you have strength, willpower, purpose, and a strong sense of self. When it is blocked, you experience fear and anxiety, as well as the proverbial "butterflies in the stomach." If you're feeling disempowered, if you're in an emotionally abusive relationship, or if you're stuck or lacking purpose in your life, this chakra will most definitely be blocked. Likewise, it is often blocked if either your first or second chakra are blocked. It's hard to feel powerful if you are feeling insecure, unstable, or sexually shut down.

The fourth chakra, called the **Heart chakra**, is in the middle of your chest, not where your anatomical heart lives. The heart center is about love and connection. There is a direct relationship between your heart chakra and your second chakra. Often, if your heart chakra is closed, your sexuality will also be shut down. Conversely, when your heart is open, it's much easier to access your sexual center. The heart chakra is also the bridge between the lower and upper chakras and connects your lower physical energy chakras with your higher spiritual energy chakras. Heart chakras can be blocked for many reasons, including:

- Protecting yourself from being emotionally hurt
- Fear of rejection
- Lack of self-love and compassion
- Grief
- Fear of being vulnerable

It's important to realize that our chakras are very flexible; they are constantly changing as we change. For example, after a recent breakup from a long-term partner, my second chakra completely shut down. I was not the least bit interested in men or sex, and I completely lost my libido. For several months, I didn't even self-pleasure because it was not a turn-on. It took me almost a year to go through my grieving process and integrate the lessons I learned from that relationship. Only then did my second chakra open and start flowing again so I could connect with another man on a sexual level.

Principles of Tantra

According to Anand:

> Tantra views the human body as a single energy phenomenon. At one end of the spectrum, at the physical level, this energy is expressed as the sex drive. At the other end of the spectrum, at the level of the nervous system and the brain, energy is experienced as ecstasy. Sexual energy is the raw material, "the crude oil," from which the high-octane fuel of ecstasy is produced. In Tantra we cultivate and move our sexual energy, which is generated in the lower chakras, into the higher chakras to help us experience a state of bliss. When a chakra is blocked, it prevents the sexual energy from flowing up the inner flute, thereby preventing us from experiencing sexual ecstasy.

There are four major Tantra principles that we use to help unblock chakras and move sexual energy:

- Breath
- Sound
- Movement
- Conscious touch

Breath is the most powerful tool that you have to unblock your chakras and feel more sensation and pleasure. It's the equivalent of putting premium gas into your car's engine. Joseph Kramer, who founded the Sexological Bodywork training, says that "the more you breathe, the more you feel." This is true on many different levels. The more oxygen you bring into your body, the more awake and alive your nerve endings become, so you feel more sensation. Breath also helps you connect with your emotions, so the more breath you bring in, the more emotions you will feel. Breath connects the energy between all of the chakra centers so that sexual energy can more easily flow.

There are many different breathing techniques we practice in Tantra, from slow deep breathing to very hard and fast breathing. Slow deep breathing is very important to help relax the body, which is critical to experiencing orgasm. Fast breathing can help increase your level of arousal. Very intense prolonged breathing can bring you to a different level of awareness and consciousness. Some of my favorite SkyDancing practices are the active meditations originally devised by Osho and later incorporated into the SkyDancing curriculum. In an active meditation, you use breath, sound, and movement, often moving around the room or in your own personal space. This allows you to truly surrender into sensation and emotions and often creates a profound meditative experience.

If breath is the premium gas that you use to charge up your chakras, then sound is next in line. Sound waves are also very powerful, because they too are a form of energy. For most women, making sounds during sex is very challenging. It's interesting how we have no problem using our voices all day long, but we freeze up when it comes to making sounds during sex. Shame has a lot to do with this, as we were socialized to believe that making deep guttural noises is somehow unladylike. Often there's also a feeling that our pleasure is private and should not be witnessed by another. But just like breath, when you make sounds, you free up some of the blocked energy in your chakras.

Exercise: Chakra Sounding

One of the easiest ways to unblock energy in your chakras is through sound vibrations. In addition to having a color and earth element, each chakra also has a corresponding sound. For this exercise, sit on the floor or a chair and make sure your feet are touching the ground. Place your right hand on your base chakra area (near the perineum) and make the deep sound "LOM." Take your time with this sound, being sure to put emphasis on both the "o" vowel and "m" sound for at least five seconds each. The longer you can hold this note, the more powerful it will be. Notice the vibration in your body and see if you can feel it in your first chakra. Now place your hand right below your belly button and make the sound "VOM." For the third chakra, place your hand below your solar plexus and say "ROM." For the fourth chakra, place your hand on your heart center and say "YOM." Then place your hand gently on your throat and make the sound "HOM." For the sixth chakra, place your hand on your third eye, which is in between your eyebrows, and say "OHM." Place your hand on the crown of your head and just listen to the internal sounds that you notice as if your ears were plugged up. A fun variation of this is to have your partner do these sound vibrations on your body while placing their mouth on or over each of the chakras.

Movement and touch are both very powerful ways to help unblock your chakras and move sexual energy. They are most effective when combined with breath and sound. Movement is a key component of SkyDancing Tantra, from dancing to rocking your pelvis during some of the breathing practices. We want to connect with our bodies since sex happens in the body, and the more connected we are, the more sensations we feel. Movement during sex also helps free up blocked energy. Moving your hips around during foreplay rather than keeping them still will help increase your level of arousal and sensations and create stronger orgasms.

Touch is another important tool we use to unblock the chakras. Touch alone can be very healing since it releases oxytocin (the cuddle hormone). Even touching yourself lovingly will increase your oxytocin levels. I can often help release energy from a client's blocked chakra just by touching it and giving it some attention. If you are sensitive to subtle energy, you can feel heat coming out of a chakra as the energy starts to move. If the chakra is totally blocked, it may feel cold. Touching your body during sex, especially your breasts, belly, arms, and legs, will help to distribute sensation and move some of the energy that may be stuck in your genitals to other parts of your body. This will free up orgasm and also increase the amount of sensation and pleasure you can experience.

If all of this talk about Tantra intrigues you, please go take a class. Tantra is almost impossible to learn just from reading a book or watching a video. It's very experiential, and you learn a lot from seeing demonstrations and being in the group energy. I highly recommend the SkyDancing Tantra workshops offered by the Ecstatic Living Institute, where I teach, or any class taught by Margot Anand. If you want to learn very specific techniques and skills (G-spot massage, prostate massage), take a class from Charles Muir at the Source School of Tantra. There are other excellent Tantra teachers around the US and internationally. For more recommendations, check the Resources section at the end of the book.

Chapter 11

HOW TO REIGNITE YOUR SHRINKING LIBIDO

As we talked about in Chapter 3, one of the most common complaints among women is loss of interest in sex. This complaint is universal, regardless of age or hormonal status. Married women, single women, newlyweds, new moms, premenopausal and postmenopausal women—all come to me on a regular basis when they no longer feel sexual desire. The fact that we are preprogrammed to say "no" to sex is one of the underlying causes of this, but it is not the only one. Since an orgasmic life requires us to be sexually alive and awake, it's important to understand some of the other reasons women lose their desire for sex. This chapter will also address ways to revive your interest in this vital part of life that can nourish you on so many levels.

Desire and Your Hormones

One issue that needs to be addressed up front is how women's hormones and cycles play into our desire and libido. From a purely biological perspective, a woman's level of estrogen has a powerful influence on her desire for sex. We know that our estrogen level peaks right before ovulation and begins dropping after ovulation until we start to menstruate, and then the cycle starts over again. Some women experience an increase in desire right around the middle of their cycle, which is Mother Nature's way of encouraging us to procreate. However, this is definitely not a universal experience. Plenty of women do not notice changes in their level of desire during the various stages of their menstrual cycle.

Hormones can definitely play havoc with your body, including your sexual desire, especially anytime they fluctuate greatly, such as during pregnancy, perimenopause, and menopause. The use of hormonal birth control, especially progesterone, can also cause significant fluctuations in your hormones and therefore in your sexual desire. I have worked with several women whose libido came back after going off the pill. I have also worked with women who experienced no impact on their libido from birth control pills. In the same vein, I have seen women whose sex drive increased during pregnancy and those whose libido dropped. The same is true of women going through menopause: some become more interested in sex, others lose interest altogether. Some women get a libido boost from supplemental estrogen or testosterone while others are not impacted at all. I do suggest that you have your hormones checked if you are experiencing low libido for more than six months, as hormone adjustments and supplements could be beneficial for you.

My point here is that women's desire and our libido is multifaceted and complex. The pharmaceutical industry has invested billions of dollars in research and development to try to find the female version of Viagra but so far has come up short. The FDA approved the pill "Addy" in 2015, but it only works in 50 percent of women, has to be taken on a daily basis, messes with your brain chemistry, and has significant side effects. Most experts are very doubtful that there will ever be a "magic pill" that women can take to increase their desire because female sexual arousal and desire are so different than that of our male counterparts. A pill simply cannot ameliorate all of the many complex factors that impact women's desire.

Desire and Your Internal Landscape

When we talk about women's libido, we need to look at both the internal and external landscapes. "Internal landscape" refers to your emotional state of being, since your emotions have a huge impact on your sexual desire. Whenever a woman comes to me complaining about low desire, one of the first questions that I ask is what's going on in her relationship, if she has one. Very frequently, decreased desire is directly related to underlying issues in a relationship such as anger, resentment, and mistrust. Sexual problems in a relationship are often the symptom, not the real problem. It makes total sense since sex for women is much more about the emotional connection than the actual physical act. Naturally, when we are feeling emotionally disconnected from our partner because we have built up anger or resentment, we have no desire to have sex.

This feeling and loss of desire can last for an extended period of time, even decades, as was the case in my marriage. If relationship issues are one of the root causes, it's unlikely your desire and sex life will improve until those relationship issues are addressed and you feel more emotionally connected with your partner. If there's been a breach of trust in the relationship, especially if one of the partners has been cheating, repairing the trust can take a long time. In my work with couples, we generally spend a significant amount of time repairing and strengthening the relationship and recreating emotional intimacy before working on the issue of sex. Often the desire to have sex comes back quickly after the emotional connection has been reestablished.

Even if the relationship is solid, unexpressed emotions can prevent you from feeling sufficiently connected with your partner to want to have sex. Something as small as being angry that your partner didn't take out the garbage or as big as a tragic loss can create blocks to intimacy. The more skilled you become at expressing your feelings, the less likely you are to shut down sexually when you feel anger or resentment. Remember that there is a direct energetic connection between your emotional heart and your sexuality. For them both to operate at an optimal level, they both need to be open and cleared of any blocks.

SkyDancing Tantra teaches us how to clear the emotional body before making love or having another type of physical connection. We become intentional about the experience we want by creating Sacred Space.

Exercise: Sacred Space Ritual: A Partner Practice

This is used with permission from the Ecstatic Living Institute's Timeless Loving™ Workshop. Please note that this is a shortened version of the Sacred Space Ritual.

Start by eliminating all potential distractions, including phones, TV, pets, or children. Set at least an hour aside just to connect with each other and be present. Two hours is ideal.

1. Sit across from each other on a bed or on the floor. It's nice to sit on a special blanket or sarong that you only use during Tantric practice. It helps signify that you are entering into a special ritual.

2. Each of you place your hands together and gently bow to each other acknowledging and thanking your partner for engaging in this ritual with you.

3. Use your hands to create an imaginary bubble around the both of you, making sure to seal it up tight. This bubble demarks a container that only the two of you inhabit. The bubble and sacred space move with you wherever you go (the hot tub, shower, bedroom, etc.) It does not leave you until you pop it at the end of your intimate time.

4. Take turns taking things out of the bubble that will not be helpful for your time together. You may only take your own things out, not your partner's, and you are not allowed to discuss these things or question your partner. This is where we get rid of emotional congestion. State out loud what you are each taking out. Examples include "distractions," "not being focused," "being tired," "being upset about our fight this morning," "the kids waking up," "your in-laws," etc. Continue until each of you feels complete. It's perfectly

fine if one partner has more or less to take out of the bubble than the other partner.

5. Now take turns bringing into the bubble the qualities/experiences you want, such as "connection," "love," "sexiness," "playfulness," "vulnerability," "honesty," etc.

6. Take turns giving each other three compliments, stating specifically what you appreciate about your partner. You can compliment his/her physical attributes ("I love how your eyes twinkle when I look into them"), other qualities ("You have such a big heart"), or specific actions ("It was so great how you helped our neighbors shovel their snow"). The more specific you are, the more solidly the appreciation will land.

7. Take turns stating your desires, fears, and boundaries for whatever activity you may be engaging in. In addition to doing this ritual before lovemaking, I often recommend it to couples who are getting over a fight, feel disconnected, or need to have an important conversation. When stating your desires, fears, and boundaries, be sure that you are only talking about your own desires and not projecting on your partner. It's fine to say, "My desire is that you touch me all over my body with a feather." It's not OK to say, "My desire is that you don't touch me in the horrible way you touched me last time we had sex." Most of us find it a bit challenging to set boundaries, even more so with an intimate partner. Some people feel uncomfortable talking about what's okay and not okay. Others aren't even aware that they have boundaries or only become aware when a boundary is crossed. You can set boundaries about time, parts of your body you don't want touched, or activities you don't want to engage in. For example, "Please stay away from my breasts today because they are really tender."

8. When the activity or conversation is complete, come back together, and facing one another, bow and intentionally put your fingers up in the air and pop the imaginary bubble.

Vanilla Sex Can Kill Your Libido

Another part of our internal landscape that contributes to low libido is boredom. As discussed in Chapter 3, boredom goes hand in hand with not experiencing enough pleasure during sex. Many couples describe their sex as "vanilla," meaning it's conventional, typically missionary position, and rote. You know what I mean by rote: same kind of foreplay every time, standard one or two positions, all very predictable and safe. This happens because we get into a routine in our sex life just as we get into routines in the rest of our lives. Humans are creatures of habit, and unfortunately, sex is no exception. When sex becomes boring and you're not having enough pleasure, watching the newest episode of *Game of Thrones* becomes a higher priority than having sex.

Boring Sex: Karen's Story

Karen came to see me because she had lost her desire to have sex with Kevin, who she completely adored and had been with for over fifteen years. They had a great relationship—except for the sex. Karen told me sex was boring; Kevin wasn't turning her on, and she felt she'd rather be chatting with her friends on Facebook. When we talked about her past sexual experiences, it became apparent that she'd had lots of wild and unconventional sex before marriage. Kevin was much more conservative. His idea of wild sex was doggie style rather than the missionary position. Karen wanted more unconventional sex with Kevin but was afraid to bring it up. She feared that if he knew about her past sexual exploits, he would lose respect for her and label her as a slut. Karen had shut down the more adventurous side of her sexuality when she met Kevin. It is not surprising that she quickly became bored with sex. This is a prime example of how the Madonna/

Whore complex shows up for women. It was fine for Karen to be the "Whore" when she was single, but the minute the marrying type came along, she felt she had to turn into the "Madonna."

I worked with Karen and Kevin and helped them navigate conversations about what they each desired in their sex life and how it could be improved. Much to Karen's surprise (but not mine), Kevin was thrilled and titillated with Karen's desire to spice things up. He loved her idea of playing with some light bondage using ropes and blindfolds. He even got into some role-playing. Last time I talked to Karen she said, "I created a monster!" Apparently, Kevin took the task of spicing up their sex life to heart, and they now have a whole closetful of toys, books, instructional videos, and costumes for fantasy play.

Desire and Your External Landscape

Your external landscape is composed of all of the external circumstances that impact your desire. This ranges from environmental conditions, such as being on vacation, being free of kids, the sights, sounds, and smells of a room, and what you are wearing to what's happening in the moment. You might notice that your desire for sex changes if after you've been wined and dined, your partner draws you a hot bath, puts on sensual music, and then welcomes you into a candlelit room filled with beautiful aromas and a bed topped with soft, silky sheets. Or maybe what turns you on is being dominated or taken by your partner in a more sexually aggressive way.

When we look at some of the factors that impact your external landscape, inability to communicate with your partner about your sex life and your needs and desires is a very common problem.

Poor communication around sex can be due to a number of reasons. First, it may just be symptomatic of other communication problems in your relationship. If you feel that you are not being heard, that your opinions are not important, and that your needs are not being met outside of the bedroom, there's no way that it's going to happen successfully within the bedroom. But let's assume you're in a solid relationship with good communication, except when it comes to sex. More often than not, the culprit that gets in the way of honest and open communication is shame (there's that five-letter word again).

Karen was ashamed to tell her husband what she wanted in bed, fearing that she would be judged as a "loose woman." Of course, the best way to normalize shame is to talk about it. When I work with couples where shame is an issue in their sex life, we have a "shame-a-thon" session wherein the partners take turns revealing their most shameful sexual experiences, thoughts, and desires. This is incredibly powerful because it creates connection and empathy, neutralizes the shame, and opens couples up to a new level of intimacy. If this is something you struggle with in your relationship, try doing the Sexual Blueprint Exercise in Chapter 4 with your partner.

To better understand your desire and the relationship between your internal and external landscape, let's look at one of your peak sexual experiences. Some of us may feel as if we have never had a peak sexual experience, and that is completely normal. If that applies to you, then complete this exercise using the best sexual experience you've had to date.

Exercise: Peak Sexual Experience

Think back over all your sexual encounters with other people. Allow your mind to focus on one or two encounters that were among the most arousing of your entire life. Try not to judge these encounters. Being turned on by what you may perceive as a "negative" feeling in a sexual encounter is completely acceptable.

1. Describe the encounter in as much detail as possible. Describe the location, objects around you, colors you remember, sounds, smells, sensations.

2. How old were you when this happened?

3. What kind of relationship did you have with the partner(s) in this encounter?

   a. Anonymous
   b. Acquaintance
   c. Boyfriend/girlfriend
   d. Primary relationship or spouse
   e. Multiple partners
   f. Other (specify)

4. What do you think made this encounter so exciting?

5. On a scale of 1–5, (where one is the least and five is the most) how would you rate your level of excitement during this encounter, especially compared to your usual ones?

6. On a scale of 1–5, how would you rate your level of fulfillment?

7. On a scale of 1–5, how important was each of the following six groups of emotions in the encounter? Within each group of feelings, base your rating on whichever feeling was most important. (Note: some emotions, especially the "negative" ones, may be very important even though they are not particularly intense).

a. Exuberance (related emotions: joy, celebration, surprise, freedom, euphoria, and pride)

b. Satisfaction (related emotions: contentment, happiness, relaxation, and security)

c. Closeness (related emotions: love, tenderness, affection, connection, oneness, and appreciation)

d. Anxiety (related emotions: fear, vulnerability, weakness, worry, and nervousness)

e. Guilt (related emotions: remorse, naughtiness, dirtiness, and shame)

f. Anger (related emotions: hostility, contempt, hatred, resentment, and revenge)

What did you notice as a result of this exercise? What did you learn about the intersection between your inner landscape and emotions and the external environment? Was this exercise challenging for you? Did you judge yourself or your peak sexual experience? Don't worry if you feel like you've never had a peak sexual experience. Later on, we are going to look at what a peak sexual experience might look like for you.

Knowing What You Want

Women also lose their libido when they are not getting what they want. The problem is that many women don't have a clue what they want. They just know that what they are getting is not doing it for them. What's more, a lot of women don't even know what else there *is* to want, sexually speaking. Rare is the woman who looks at porn or searches for sex tips and techniques online. And if she did, she would still have to figure out how to ask for what she wants sexually without the fear of possibly ruffling her partner's feathers.

Consider for a moment what you're not getting from your partner during sex. If you are like most women, your unmet needs fall into several different but related categories:

- You don't feel emotionally connected
- You don't like the way your partner touches you
- You are not getting enough foreplay
- You don't like the way your partner initiates physical intimacy

- You don't feel desired
- You aren't sure your partner is attracted to you

Remember: Women need to feel an emotional connection with their partners in order to desire sex. This is the number one need and the one that is most often not met. If you want more sex and intimacy, first make sure the emotional connection is solid. Let's focus on some other needs that are not met during sex.

If you don't like the way your partner touches you, you are not alone. This is the most frequent complaint I hear from women.

- Touch that is too fast, too hard, too soft, too rough
- Touch that feels like your partner has an agenda
- Being touched too soon on your breasts or pussy
- Touch without kissing
- Annoying, repetitive touch that makes you feel like your partner is not really present

Women are not getting enough foreplay. In a recent survey of 500 women by fertility app Kindara, when questioned "What makes sex good?" 56 percent of women said an emotional connection and 23 percent said enough foreplay. But how much foreplay are we getting? Five to nine minutes, according to a 2008 survey of 1,000 women by *Glamour* magazine.[13] Those numbers are consistent with government-funded studies. Five to nine minutes is barely enough time for a woman to reach even a low level of arousal. Most women need thirty to forty-five minutes of foreplay before they are aroused enough for penetration to be pleasurable!

---

13 Glamour.com. "How Many Minutes Sex and Foreplay Really Last," Glamour Magazine, 2008. https://www.glamour.com/story/how-many-minutes-sex-and-forep.

Premature penetration prevents women from enjoying sex, because they don't have access to higher levels of pleasure and orgasm.

Who Initiates Sex?

Does it ever bother you that sex is always initiated by the same person? Or maybe you wish that the way sex was initiated could be more exciting or interesting. Many women are turned off when their partner hints that they want sex. It could be bad timing, or you might be totally exhausted and stressed out. It makes sex feel more like an obligation than a desire. How sex is initiated is important for you to feel turned on. Foreplay starts long before you touch. For example, sending teasing, flirty text messages builds up anticipation, creates tension, and is a great way to initiate a romantic encounter.

"I don't feel like my partner wants to have sex with me or is attracted to me anymore." I hear this from both men and women. This often comes up in conversations around how sex is initiated. Not feeling desired makes us feel unattractive and not sexy, which is one of the quickest ways to shut us down sexually. It's a turn-on for most women to feel desired. It brings out our sexy self and helps connect us with our sexual power. Most women also relate desire to passion, which is another need that is often not met by our partners.

Understand Your Sexual Style

How do we begin to get our needs met? Let's start with figuring out what your sexual style is. One of the many reasons that couples struggle in the bedroom is that they have different sexual styles. Sexual styles were first articulated by the psychologist Donald

Mosher and popularized by David Schnarch[14] in his bestselling book *Passionate Marriage: Keeping Love and Intimacy Alive in Committed Relationships*.

There are three types of sexual styles:

- Trance State
- Partner Engagement
- Role-Play and Fantasy[15]

We all have a primary sexual style, although you may be able to move between some or all of them. Read the following descriptions and see if you can figure out what your primary sexual style is. As an added bonus, figure out your partner's sexual style.

Trance State: If you are someone who likes to close your eyes, go inside, and really focus on physical sensation, you are a "trancer." You are likely highly kinesthetic, meaning that touch is the primary way in which you connect with a partner during lovemaking. Trancers tend to like very slow, focused touch. You need minimal distractions; even the slightest interruption can short-circuit your arousal. You can go very deep and even have an out-of-body experience during sex. Emotional connection may be more difficult to maintain because your focus is on your own pleasure rather than on your partner.

Partner Engagement: If sex is about emotion, romance, lots of kissing and eye contact, your sexual style is partner engagement. Intimacy and connection is most important for this style. You like to be romanced with tender, loving words. You need to be in the right mood and a pleasing atmosphere. Partner Engagers tend to shy away from casual sexual encounters.

---

14 Check out his site: http://passionatemarriage.com/

15 David Schnarch, *Passionate Marriage: Keeping Love and Intimacy Alive in Committed Relationships*. W.W. Norton & Co., Reprint Edition, 2009. Print.

Role-Play and Fantasy: If you are someone who needs to go into a fantasy in order to get really aroused during sex, or if sex for you is about role-play, then this is your sexual style. This style involves a lot of creativity and exploration and the ability and breadth to play many different roles. Role-playing in particular requires a fair degree of comfort with your own individuality and sexual expression.

When Sexual Styles Conflict

When partners in a relationship have different sexual styles, conflicts can arise that impact their intimate life in a variety of ways. You may feel like your partner becomes distant during sex, literally disappearing inside of themselves. Or maybe you are frustrated because sex isn't that satisfying for you. Physical cues are easily misinterpreted. You like eye contact during sex and feel abandoned when your partner closes their eyes. Fantasy helps to get you aroused, but it makes you feel guilty. All your partner hears is "blame" that they are not doing something right. But it's not their fault. You don't understand how your sexual style impacts your arousal.

Conflicting Sexual Styles: Anne and Jeremy's Story

Anne and Jeremy came to see me because Anne was no longer attracted to Jeremy. While there were several issues impacting her desire, one of them was related to the conflict in their sexual styles. Anne's sexual style was trance; she felt most comfortable going inside and having her eyes closed during sex. Jeremy's style was partner engagement. He liked to keep his eyes open during sex. Anne often felt that his energy was "too big," and she got very uncomfortable when he initiated sex. Here was the perfect storm.

Jeremy was being triggered when Anne closed her eyes while making love, because to him it felt like she was disengaged and emotionally detached. Anne was getting triggered when Jeremy kept his eyes open while making love, because to her, his insistent eye contact was intrusive and caused her to feel overwhelmed by his "big energy."

I worked with Anne and Jeremy to help them understand each other's sexual styles. We talked at length about what they each needed during lovemaking to feel connected and safe. Anne learned that she could open her eyes during sex, take little glances at Jeremy, and go back to her trance state. This made Jeremy feel more connected to her. Jeremy learned how to lessen the intensity of his energy and back off a bit on the eye contact. He found a whole new level of connection with Anne when he relaxed into himself and watched her enjoy her state of trance.

Switching it Up: Sexual Styles Aren't Static

Sexual styles are fluid. You can switch it up, intentionally or unintentionally. You can go back and forth between them and try out different styles with full awareness—or not. In fact, most of us discover our sexual style through experimentation, so why not experiment with clear intent? You might be surprised at what you discover.

I switch back and forth between partner engagement and trance state. During foreplay, I like to engage with my partner and feel our connection through eye contact and some sexy talk. Once I'm feeling emotionally connected and we've established safety, I switch into a trance state. I feel much more sensation in my body when my eyes are closed and I'm not visually distracted. I stay in trance state for intercourse and orgasmic play, although I will often open my eyes and take small glances at my partner so he knows I am still there. When I am with a new partner, I tend to stay in trance state during our initial foreplay as we establish a level of intimacy and comfort, then I can switch over to partner engagement.

Knowing your sexual style is important to getting your needs met. Equally important is understanding your sexual desires and fantasies, which can help you achieve a peak sexual experience.

Core Erotic Theme

In the book, *The Erotic Mind: Unlocking the Inner Source of Passion and Fulfillment*, Jack Morin discusses the concept of a "core erotic theme." A core erotic theme consists of the people, images, and experiences that turn you on and are the most arousing. The core erotic theme always has a direct connection with our past challenges and difficulties. The core erotic theme is often a direct reflection of a past challenge that can be recreated under different circumstances. Rape victims often have a core erotic theme involving a rape fantasy, except they are in control of the scene. Or the core erotic theme can show up as the exact opposite of one of your core childhood wounds.[16]

Your core erotic theme plays a major role in sexual desire. Your fantasies, desires, and peak sexual experiences comprise your core erotic theme. If you can express your core erotic theme during sex, you will be able to feel more desire and arousal, which will lead you toward more orgasmic life force energy. The turn-on is not necessarily from the act itself, but rather from the emotions and feelings behind the action. For example, my core erotic

16 Jack Morin, *The Erotic Mind*. Harper Collins, 1995. Print.

theme is about being defenseless and completely at someone else's mercy. My fantasies tend to involve being caged, tied up, and on public display. During sex, huge turn-ons for me include having my hair pulled, my arms being restrained, or feeling dominated in some way. My childhood experiences of being both defenseless in the face of my father's death and having to rely on myself play right into my core erotic theme. For someone who is fiercely independent, submission is freedom. I get turned on when I'm bound up, blindfolded, and told to obey instructions. When someone else is in control, I get to let go of my tendency to micromanage situations and completely surrender to desire.

To explore your core erotic theme, we're going to borrow a page from *Making Love Real* by Celeste Hirschman and Danielle Harel and examine what they call your "hottest sexual movie." Essentially, we all have a unique "sexual movie" that turns us on and expresses our core erotic theme. Hirschman and Harel identify four basic themes to these movies that drive the plot, if you will. They are:

- The Romantic Movie (think *Titanic*)
- The Passionate Movie (unbridled passion)
- The Dominant/Submissive Movie (think *Secretary*)
- The Spiritual Movie (Goddess worship)[17]

If you're like me, you can probably step in and play a role in any one of these movies. You might even have a favorite that always gets you where you want to go. But what we're looking for in this exercise is the one that really rings your bell. Once you know that, you will have identified your true core erotic theme.

---

17 Celeste Hirschman and Danielle Harel, *Making Love Real*. Somatica Press, 2015. Print.

EXERCISE: IDENTIFYING YOUR HOTTEST SEXUAL MOVIE

Examine the themes in each of these movies. Review the phrases below and notice which ones you resonate with. Make a list of all those phrases and any others that occur to you. Share with a partner how you define each of these movies (e.g., what does romance mean to you, and how do you want to be romanced) and the phrases that you would like a partner to use for each of these movies. Then practice with each other because these phrases may feel foreign in the beginning.

Romantic Movie: This movie is about being deeply cared for and loved. It is the most common movie in our culture. It embodies the Cinderella fantasy.

- Timeless attraction: "You are the most beautiful woman I've ever seen."
- Preciousness: "Being close to you means more to me than anything else in the world."
- The one and only: "I've never loved someone the way I've loved you."
- Physical appreciation: "You are so beautiful." "You smell so good."

Passionate Movie: This movie is about animalistic, intense, insatiable desire.

- Tell them what you want to do to them: "I could spend hours licking and teasing you."
- Share the intensity of your physical need: "I want you to be inside me right now."
- Share how strongly you feel about them: "When you touch me, I get a chill running through my body and feel myself getting wet."
- Talk about how much they delight you: "I love the sounds you make when you come."

Dominant/Submissive Movie: A very common movie is about power. It may be that you are powerless (submissive) or that you are in control (dominant).

- Command: "Spread your legs." "Get on all fours."
- Revoke permission: "Did I tell you it was OK to look at me? Look at the ground."
- Praise: "You've been a very good girl."
- Punish/degrade: "You're a dirty little slut."
- Disapprove: "I told you to stick your tongue inside of me. Is that as far as you can go?"
- Possess: "That pussy is mine! I'll tell you when you can touch it." "You belong to me, and I will do with you as I please."

The Spiritual Movie: This movie is often about worshipping the goddess. It is played out more in creating the atmosphere around sexuality rather than with phrases: candles, essential oils, creating sacred space, eye gazing, and connecting with breath. A woman receives pleasure from her partner and can choose whether to give back or just enjoy the experience of being worshipped. Tantric rituals may also be included, helping to create a spiritual connection with your partner.

Write down what really turns you on and the feelings and emotions your movie evokes. Try not to judge yourself. Often some of our most arousing feelings and emotions are the most challenging and uncomfortable. They are definitely worth exploring.

Now that you understand more about your core erotic theme and hottest sexual movie, consider what would it take to have some of that in your sex life. When you know what you want, it's a whole lot easier to get your needs met.

In the next chapter, we are going to discuss the issue of sexual polarity between partners. It is one of the most important aspects of creating a healthy and juicy sex life and has a huge impact on women's libido.

Chapter 12

SEXUAL POLARITY: WHAT MOST WOMEN CRAVE

Why Opposites Attract

For most women, one of the factors that makes for hot, passionate sex is sexual polarity in the relationship. It is true that opposites attract each other. The sexual charge that shows up when we're having passionate sex occurs because of the tension between masculine and feminine energy. When there is a lot of sexual polarity with your partner, the charge is strong. When that doesn't exist, sex might be nice and sweet, but lacks the passion that you really want. Think about a battery: positive to negative conducts a charge, positive to positive or negative to negative does not. Few have explained this concept better than David Deida in his internationally renowned book, *The Way of the Superior Man*.

> Sexual attraction is based upon sexual polarity, which is the force of passion that arcs between the masculine and feminine poles…[thus] creating the flow of sexual feeling. This force of attraction, which flows between the two different poles of masculine and feminine, is the dynamism that often disappears in the modern relationship. If you want real passion, you need a ravisher and a ravishee, otherwise

you just have two buddies who rub genitals in bed.... The love may still be strong, the friendship may still be strong, but the sexual polarity fades unless in moments of intimacy one partner is willing to play the masculine pole and one partner is willing to play the feminine. You have to animate the masculine and the feminine differences if you want to play in the field of sexual passion.[18]

In the world of Tantra, we often refer to sexual energy as either being Yang (pronounced "Yong") or Yin. The Yang energy has qualities that we traditionally consider to be more masculine: strength, hardness, patience, achievement, persistence, and perfection. The Yin energy has more traditional feminine qualities: expressiveness, beauty, receptivity, surrender, softness, and flow. You have both Yin feminine and Yang masculine energy inside of you. The degree to which you've cultivated these two energies varies from person to person. For example, there are men who hold a lot of masculine energy (Bruce Willis) but haven't cultivated their softer, feminine side. There are also men (Canada's Prime Minister Justin Trudeau, President Obama) who have cultivated more of their feminine side. Similarly, there are women (Rachel Maddow, Hillary Clinton) who hold strong male energy and others (Princess Di, Marilyn Monroe) whose energy is primarily feminine.

When I work with heterosexual couples to help them find their sexual polarity, I am often asked, "Does this mean that the male partner has to be the dominant masculine energy?" I tell them, "Definitely not, as long as one of the partners plays the masculine energy role." There are many happy couples in which the woman plays the dominant role to a more submissive male

---

18 David Deida, *The Way of the Superior Man: A Spiritual Guide to Mastering the Challenges of Women, Work, and Sexual Desire*. Plexus Press, Austin, TX, 1997.

partner. Also, you can easily switch back and forth between playing the masculine and feminine energy roles. It should also be noted that this is not true for all couples. Just as there is no "one size fits all" way to have sex, there is also no "one size fits all" approach to what turns us on or turns us off.

In our society, sexual polarity is nonexistent in many long-term relationships. I often hear couples complain that they miss the spark they felt in the beginning of the relationship. That spark, new relationship energy, is different than sexual polarity, although it feels the same. In her book, *Why We Love: The Nature and Chemistry of Romantic Love*, researcher Helen Fisher examined what happens to our brains in the early stages of love. The euphoria, excitement, and rush that we feel are related to shifts in our brain chemistry. Dopamine (the addiction hormone) increases, as does norepinephrine (the high energy "rush" hormone). These hormones light up the amygdala, the pleasure center in the brain, causing us to crave more connection, contact with our partner, and sex. An important outcome of this phase is that it helps us to form secure attachments. The challenge is that soon, in anywhere from six to eighteen months, the new relationship energy vanishes, and the sexual charge often disappears as well. The lack of that passion can play havoc with your desire.[19]

One of the best ways to bring passion back into a relationship is to teach men how to cultivate their strong masculine sexual side so that women can surrender into our softer feminine side. The true nature of the feminine is to surrender into the strong, masculine sexual energy. In fact, many women actually enjoy being physically dominated, taken, and ravished by a man. It is important to note that this is a conscious choice made by the woman in each

19 Helen E. Fisher, *Why We Love: The Nature and Chemistry of Romantic Love*. New York: Henry Holt and, 2005.

instance to differentiate the fantasy from the real act of violence and violation that happens in rape or nonconsensual touch.

Fantasy and Cultural Taboos

Daniel Bergner speaks to this in his book, *What Do Women Want? Adventures in the Science of Female Desire*. He draws from his interviews with women about their fantasies and reports on more than a dozen studies on women's sexual desire and arousal. Bergner found that "rape fantasy" was one of the most common fantasies for women. Rape fantasies involved either physical force, the threat of force, or any nonconsensual sexual activity, including sleep or intoxication. Bergner found that between 30–60 percent of women fantasized about this type of sexual activity during sex, masturbation, and daydreaming. The researchers involved in these studies believe that the numbers are probably higher but are underreported, given women's shame around this issue.[20]

Let's be clear. A rape fantasy is completely different than actual rape, which is a brutal act of violence. There are very few women who have been raped who actually fantasize about it after the fact. The researchers Bergner interviewed believe that the rape fantasy helps women escape from sexual shame we harbor from early childhood. Imagining and relishing a rape fantasy breaks a taboo, as a part of some women's core erotic themes. Also, a fantasy allows us to control the stimuli; in actual rape, there is no control. At its heart, a rape fantasy is about submission, being dominated and taken by a man or a group of men. For many women, it's a huge turn-on to feel that their partner desires them so much that the partner is willing to overpower them.

20 Daniel Bergner, *What Do Women Want? Adventures in the Science of Female Desire*. Harper Collins, 2014.

My own "research" with women around this desire to be taken is consistent with Bergner's. In my Passionate Intimacy workshop for couples, I ask the women in the room, "Who would be turned on if your partner threw you up against the wall and started to ravish you?" Without fail, every female hand in the room shoots up while the men stand around in the room with mouths agape.

Bergman also reports that many of his interviewees' fantasies were of having wild sex with the rogue man...the bad boy. The "good guys" are for relationships and dating, but not for having intense, passionate sex. I asked men at my Master Lover Workshop to describe a "bad boy." "Doesn't treat a woman well," said one man. "Disrespectful and sexually aggressive," said another. "Violates boundaries," said a third as all the heads nodded. They couldn't understand why women are attracted to them. The truth is we don't want to be in relationships with bad boys, they just spell trouble. But we like to have sex with bad boys because bad boys hold strong masculine energy. That creates the polarity where we find attraction, chemistry, and sexual charge.

The problem with the good guys we want as partners is that they have been socialized to be good guys with respect to sex as well. They are polite, don't cross boundaries, and ask permission for a kiss rather than reading a woman's body language. They give us sweet, gentle caresses when we're craving unbridled passionate touch. Too much gentle nurturing touch can be a turn-off for you and your partner.

Creating Sexual Polarity through Role-Play: Collette and Liam's Story

Collette and Liam were sitting in the front row of my "Men's Lover Workshop." She was tearing up the whole time. She pulled me aside afterwards and told me, "We've been engaged for eight years. I love Liam in so many ways, but our sex life is horrible. I'm not sure I can marry him." They soon became regular clients. Collette told me in a private session that one of her best sexual experiences had been being ravished by a former lover. The ravishment had the element of surprise and dominance, allowing her to surrender to pleasure. Clearly sexual polarity was not an issue in that relationship.

Things were different, though, with Liam. They were best friends and adored each other. He was attracted to her and very turned on by Collette. But she was not turned on by Liam. She complained about everything—from the way he touched her to the way he kissed her. She really struggled to feel sexual with him, and it was tearing them apart. They were clearly stuck in the "friend zone," a dangerous place to be in a long-term relationship. While Liam's skills had definitely improved, he had a hard time tapping into his more masculine Yang side, a common issue among good guys. Liam found that masculine side through a role-play exercise. He created a new persona, a sexy, seductive, confident man based on the James Bond character. He even added a costume to the role. In that role, Liam could leave his sweet, gentle side behind, and embody a more powerful and sexually dominant man. Collette loved this new side of Liam, and they are now happily married and having passionate sex.

Sexual Polarity is Upside Down in our Society

At this point you might be thinking, "Oh, no problem. We will just create the sexual polarity that you've described and our sex will become passionate again." I wish it were that easy. The power dynamics between men and women in our society are evolving. Successful, powerful women hold so much masculine energy that they find it difficult to cultivate their feminine sexual energy. Men are feeling disempowered and confused about how to exert their masculinity. Women want men to be both emotionally vulnerable and sexually dominant. It's a tall order that can leave a man scratching his head and wondering, "How do I need to show up for her to desire me sexually?"

This shift has happened gradually over the last thirty years with the rise of the feminist movement. Feminism has been a godsend for women's sexuality. There is no doubt that without the likes of Betty Friedan and Gloria Steinem, just to name a few, we would not have the sexual liberation and freedom that we currently enjoy. The feminist movement also is largely responsible for equal pay, securing civil rights, and legalizing same-sex unions. Feminism has allowed women to embrace more personal power, and in so doing, has redefined what it means to be a woman. Men in turn have been required (oftentimes reluctantly and with trepidation) to redefine masculinity in response to women's changing roles at home and in the workplace. This shift in traditional masculine and feminine roles can have a strong impact on our sense of self-worth. For both genders, questions about dependence and independence, income potential, decision-making, childrearing, etc., have become more complex.

More women attend college than men (57 to 43 percent), and women also outnumber men in most professional schools (law, medicine, veterinary). Men are increasingly leaving high school and going straight into the workforce (e.g., construction, technology, military), creating a gap between highly educated women and less educated white- and blue-collar men. The gender income gap is also at a historic low. The PEW Research Foundation reports that women now earn $0.83 for every $1 earned by a man. In 1980, it was $0.64. Millennial women (ages twenty-five to thirty-four) make 90 percent of what their male counterparts earn.

While this development is mostly positive and is a welcome change from the prescribed and narrow gender roles that our parents grew up with, it has also unwittingly impacted our sex lives. I discussed this in a 2014 article that I wrote for Elephant Journal, entitled, "How the Feminist Movement Screwed Up Our Sex Lives and What We Can Do About It."

My article was based on a book by Deborah Spar, President of Barnard College in New York City, *Wonder Woman: Sex, Power and the Quest for Perfection*. What Deborah so masterfully conveyed was the "Wonder Woman syndrome" from a historical perspective. In a nutshell: by the time girls born in the '60s and '70s entered womanhood, we'd seen a number of changes in society that had considerable impact on our lives:

- Reproductive rights secured
- Civil rights battle completed
- Vietnam War behind us
- Women's admissions to colleges and graduate school skyrocketing
- Women in the workplace in large numbers[21]

We did this without having to sign a petition, march on Washington, or burn our bras. Our mothers told us we were just as capable as men and could be whatever we aspired to be. This message was reinforced in *Ms.* magazine and popular media (think *Charlie's Angels*). One of the legacies of the feminist movement is

21 Deborah Spar, *Wonder Woman: Sex, Power and the Quest for Perfection*. Picador, 2014. Print.

that women began to believe we could have it all—a professional career, a husband, children, two cats and a dog—and keep it together.

But as I read Deborah's book, I had a powerful realization. The feminist movement began to shift the power dynamics between women and men. Women gained the opportunity to live up to the same standards of success as men. In this process, many of us had to embrace masculine values.

In my own life, I was pressured to go to law school or medical school. I chose the one that sucked the blood *out* of me. I bought into the masculine notion that success and happiness were defined by how much money I made, how big my house was, and how high I could climb on the organizational ladder. I made it all the way up to CEO, all while raising two children and keeping the family together.

Along the way, I was also taught that emotions are bad and displaying them is a weakness. I learned that screwing other people in order to get ahead in the world was not only acceptable, it was expected. Business came before pleasure and was a higher priority than spending more time with my children. I wore the pants in the family. The buck stopped with me.

And therein lies one of the reasons why many women struggle so much in our sex lives. As I rose in the business world and became more powerful and more successful, I completely lost touch with my feminine side—including my feminine sexual energy. The nurturing mother inside of me was intact, but the sexy Goddess who can surrender to passion and orgasm was nonexistent. In the process, I unwittingly further emasculated my husband, who'd already been emasculated by his domineering mother.

In the business world, I was a force to be reckoned with. Unfortunately, that force was also alive and well in the bedroom. I didn't want to be the masculine presence in the bedroom. I didn't want to be the one who always initiated sex and called the shots in my marriage. I simply never learned how to be otherwise. And it isn't only powerful businesswomen who experience this plight. Many couples struggle with the fact that women hold so much masculine energy that they have difficulty tapping into their feminine side.

Finding Her Feminine Self: Andrea's Story

Andrea, who was the forty-five-year-old CEO of her own architecture firm, was a recent divorcée whose husband had left her for another woman. Childless, Andrea was a workaholic who was married to her business and her career. The minute she walked into the room, I could sense her very obvious Yang sexual energy. Like many woman, she wanted to surrender in the bedroom, but did not know how to find her feminine self. To a control freak, surrender is not only uncomfortable but often frightening. Trusting one's partner is central to surrender.

Andrea had several blocks to work through. It was impossible for her to depend on anyone else, either at home or in business, because of childhood attachment issues. Having grown up with alcoholic parents, she became an adult who was very much responsible for her own survival. She ran away from emotional intimacy and her marriage by becoming a workaholic. After we addressed these blocks, I helped Andrea find her feminine side using some of the tools below.

Exercise: Fun Ways to Find Your Sexy

If you feel like it's hard for you to connect with your feminine side and feel sexy, try some of these activities.

- Get back into your body. Dance is one of the best ways for you to rediscover your feminine nature. Take a Salsa, tango, or ballroom dance class. Instead of kickboxing when you go to the gym, take a Zumba class. Find out if there are any Five Rhythms or Ecstatic Dance events in your area. Ecstatic Dance and Five Rhythms are freeform dance modalities with a focus on your own experience of moving your body with the music. There are no steps to follow; instead, you allow your body to follow the rhythms that you feel. Belly dancing is also a great way to get in touch with your feminine side and tone those tummy muscles in the process!

- Surround yourself with sensual things like flowers, beautiful fragrances, candles, and satin and silk.

- Start dressing sexier! Get rid of the comfy clothes that hide your body. Select some low necklines and clothes that give you some shape. Wear those Jimmy Choos! Try wearing some sexy underwear for the day and see how it makes you feel.

- Plan a girls' night out with the intent of expressing your sexy self. Go out on the town with your bestie and flirt like crazy. There's nothing like a little male attention to get your juices going again! You might even make your girls' night out a girls' night in and host a clothes swap and makeup party.

- You have to believe you're sexy to feel sexy, but for many of us, sexy is like a muscle that needs to be activated. When we ignore it, atrophy sets in. When we work it, the muscle becomes stronger. Look at yourself in the mirror and tell yourself how sexy you are.

Masculinity and Male Sexuality

Now let's look at how the shifts in power dynamics between men and women in society have been impacting men and their connection with their own sexuality. It must be really hard to be a man right now. Men are confused about exactly who they are, what they want, and how they are supposed to show up. Many men feel emasculated and disempowered in the face of strong women. And frankly, there are men who believe that women's rise to power is a serious threat to their masculinity.

When it comes to sexual dynamics, men get many mixed messages. On the one hand, we tell them, "Be more vulnerable" or, "Tap into your feminine side." On the other hand, we want to be dominated. Sexual harassment suits are on the rise, and there are even phone apps to determine whether there is true consent. No wonder men are reluctant to feel and express their desire. Men are afraid to check women out for fear of being called creepy or labeled a predator. As a result, many men are walking around completely disconnected from their sexuality and don't even feel their cocks.

Permission to Feel Desire: Paul's Story

An important part of my work with men is to give them permission to feel their desire. Paul, a recent divorcé, came to see me because he was struggling with meeting women and with the dating scene. I told Paul that we were going to do an exercise where he would be able to check me out. The thought of doing this immediately made him uncomfortable. I stood up while he was sitting on the couch and asked him to look at me from head to toe, really focusing on the parts of my body that he was not supposed to be looking at. At first, Paul could only look at my face because he wanted to be respectful. Eventually, with coaxing, Paul began looking at the rest of my body, including my breasts and my butt. Then I asked him to pretend that he was with a group of buddies and talk about my body, expressing himself as crudely as he wanted to. This was extremely hard for Paul, and he could not muster anything more than, "She's hot." Men who have been told over and over not to objectify women often end up shutting down their desire completely, even when they are given permission to express it. If you are comfortable, a great way to help your partner feel his desire and give him the permission he needs is to ask him what he would like to do to you sexually. Or invite him to check out your body and to feel his own desire build.

The current state of power dynamics between men and woman has created havoc in the bedroom. Fearful that they will cross a boundary, men hold back their desire, wanting to be the good, respectful guy, when in fact, many women crave being taken by a man. Constantly having to navigate women's shifting boundaries creates tremendous confusion for men. Men are also very sensitive to rejection and will quickly reach a point where they'd rather wait for their partner to initiate sex than face more rejection. But many women are turned off by having to initiate sex, since they also want to feel desired by their partners. This causes dysfunctional sexual relationships where no one's needs are met.

Learning to Surrender into Dominance: Genevieve and Carl's Story

Genevieve and Carl, who had been married for six years, were facing some serious challenges in their sex life. Genevieve was frustrated that she always had to initiate sex and felt her sex drive was much stronger than Carl's. Her hottest sexual movie was to be dominated and passionately taken. Before she got married, she'd had any number of lovers who had played starring roles in that movie, as had Carl in their early years. While they were both very successful in their careers, Genevieve wore the pants in the family. She often dominated Carl. The only place that Carl really felt in charge and powerful was in his office. Not surprisingly, he spent a lot of time there. Whenever Genevieve got angry with him or went on a rant, his immediate reaction was to go into a freeze state. This further frustrated Genevieve: she wanted him to take control of the situation so she didn't have to.

No surprise, then, that this same dynamic showed up in their intimacy. To help them create a better sex life, Carl had to get comfortable with dominance, which felt disrespectful to him. But before that could be effective, we had to spend many months examining and resolving the unhealthy power dynamic in their relationship, which touched both of their childhood wounds. Genevieve, who had major abandonment issues and was fiercely independent, had to learn that she could rely on Carl to take care of things in their life. Carl, who felt responsible for his parent's divorce, had to learn that when Genevieve yelled at him in anger, rather than recoiling, he actually had to reach out and soothe her and reassure her that he would not leave her. Ultimately, Carl was able to reconnect with his masculine sexual energy, and

Genevieve learned how to pull back control and allow more of her feminine energy to emerge.

If you are in a partnership, there is no question that creating more sexual polarity in the relationship will help both you and your partner access orgasmic life force energy. But one does not need to be in a relationship in order to experience orgasmic energy and lead an orgasmic life! Much of my own journey was solo, although I had lovers along the way. In the next chapter, we are going to address one of the most important ways to help you reclaim your pleasure by connecting with your own sexual energy and learning about your arousal patterns.

Chapter 13

REALIZING YOUR PLEASURE POTENTIAL

In Chapter 3, we talked about one of the primary reasons many women lose their libido: for them, sex does not equal pleasure. Women simply don't enjoy sex enough to make it a priority. Rather than feel the natural pull of desire, they go through all manner of psychological gymnastics, some of which can be quite injurious to the relationship. For example:

- You start to question whose needs are more important, "my partner's or mine?"
- You begin believing you're past your prime.
- You "give it up" even though you don't really want to have sex out of a sense of "duty."
- You blame your partner for having unrealistic expectations of sex in a long-term relationship.
- You dismiss your partner's desire and ignore their advances or deflect them with any number of excuses ("I'm too tired") or false promises ("Let's do it this weekend when the pressure is off").
- You grant your partner "mercy sex" once a month.
- You start to think your partner is a sex addict.
- In a moment of anger, you tell your partner to go ahead and have sex with someone else.

The gap between your partner's continued desire for sex and your lack of desire is a bit of a conundrum, given that your orgasmic capacity actually far exceeds his. Unlike men, women can have multiple orgasms with little or no refractory period. Under the right circumstances, each climax can take us to higher levels of pleasure and orgasmic bliss.

I use many methods to help women gain access to their orgasmic potential, some of which are drawn from Tantric principles. These tools can be learned, and with practice, can be very effective. Women who integrate these skills into their sex lives achieve levels of orgasm they have not reached before. This state of orgasmic bliss, where energy flows freely between the physical and spiritual realms, opens up the doorway to living an orgasmic life.

While I can't teach this to you in one chapter and the practices are not easy to convey in a book, I do want you to start experiencing more pleasure sooner rather than later. So let's explore a few basic principles to that end. Later in the chapter, I will share a few simple exercises that will allow you to feel more pleasure in your body right away.

Slow Things Down

Quite often, when a woman doesn't get pleasure from sex, it's because she hasn't gotten sufficiently aroused before genital contact or penetration. Most women need at least thirty to forty-five minutes of foreplay before they are ready to have sex. If you are like most couples, that is three to five times more foreplay than you are engaging in right now.

Longer foreplay means slowing everything down. In her bestselling book, *Slow Sex*, Nicole Daedone, the founder of One Taste, talks about sex as an art form rather than a science.

Like an artist in the flow of creation, we follow the experience rather than focusing on the direction we think it's supposed to go. Sex as an art form means following your desires, tuning in to your sensations, and paying attention to your body. This cannot happen if you're on automatic and "going through the motions," or if you're in a hurry to have an orgasm and get it over with.[22]

Slowing down has many benefits:

- You become more present and aware
- You build sexual energy and create sexual tension
- You create resonance with your partner, enhancing connection and intimacy
- You have access to more of your pleasure centers

Slow sex is similar to meditation, and in fact, at the core of Daedone's teaching is a practice she calls Orgasmic Meditation, or what practitioners affectionately call, "OM-ing." In a session of Orgasmic Meditation, the stroker, typically a man, strokes a certain part of the women's clitoris for fifteen minutes in a very specific way. It is one-way touch, the man uses latex gloves, he is fully clothed, and the woman is only undressed from her waist down. The woman is completely focused on her own sensation; there is no eye contact and no goal for orgasm. Men claim that the practice is meditative and helps them be more aware of their own sensations.

When you approach sexual activity as a meditation, you become much more present and in the moment. This in turn makes you much more focused and aware of everything that is happening in your body and with your partner. So many women complain

---

22 Nicole Daedone, *Slow Sex: The Art and Craft of the Female Orgasm*. New York: Grand Central Life & Style, 2012.

that their partner is not present during sex. The easiest way to become present is to slow things down.

Building sexual energy slowly generates a delicious anticipatory tension that causes you to move toward pleasure rather than away from it. Your body actually craves more touch and different types of stimulation. As you feel more desire, sexual tension increases and you come closer to having an orgasm. Creating sexual tension with your partner is not the same as the tension that you feel when you are trying too hard to have an orgasm. The latter will prevent you from coming, since orgasm happens when you are both highly aroused and highly relaxed.

Women are constantly complaining that the passion and the fire have gone out of their sex life. The remedy is simple: slow everything down, allow sexual tension to build, and allow that tension to ignite the flames of desire.

When you slow down enough to really connect with the sensations in your body and with your partner, you create resonance. Your bodies become like tuning forks. Think about it from a physics perspective. When you strike a tuning fork and set it to vibrating, a second tuning fork set at the same pitch will begin to vibrate with the first fork, emitting the same vibrational sound. The two tuning forks are connected by the surrounding air particles, which creates a sound wave. The energy created by the sound wave is tuned to the frequency of the second tuning fork, causing it to vibrate. This is called resonance, when energy moves back and forth between two or more objects.

When couples slow down, gaze into each other's eyes, and really focus on their connection, their bodies start to resonate in much the same way. You will start matching each other's breathing. Your movements begin to synchronize. This is a very powerful form of intimacy that creates the kind of emotional connection and safety that women need to enjoy sex.

Slowing things down will give you access to more of your pleasure centers, and there are many of them in your body. In the last decade, sex research has focused on the brain's involvement in sexual arousal through neuroimaging studies. Science now validates what we've known all along: every one of your five senses (sight, hearing, taste, touch, smell) is a pleasure center! And each sense perceives sexual stimulus through cues and nerve endings. The prefrontal cortex of the brain then evaluates and grades these stimuli for sex appeal. The occipital lobe causes increased attention and focus on the sexual stimulus. Signals are sent to the amygdala, the pleasure center in your brain, which is neurologically connected to the erectile tissue in your ears, nose, lips, nipples and genitals, thus causing arousal to begin.

In real life, this is how it works. If your room is filled with candles and you really take in a beautiful naked body in front of you, your eyes stimulate your arousal network. If there are essential oils, fresh fruit, or flowers, your nose will also send signals of arousal to your brain. When you hear your favorite sexy music, your ears are stimulated and send arousal signals to your brain. When you are kissed slowly, your lips and your mouth can taste the sweet kisses of your partner, sending more arousal signals to the brain. If your arms, legs, neck, and hair are slowly and lightly touched and caressed, sending chills down your body, even more arousal signals are sent to your brain. When all five senses are stimulated and firing at the same time, you will experience at least five times more sensation in your body.

Exercise: Chocogasm Meditation

One of my very favorite exercises is the Chocogasm Meditation, which takes you through the experience of awakening all of your senses as you slowly and sensually eat (or feed your partner) a piece of chocolate. All you need to have is some chocolate and ten minutes of time. If you do this exercise correctly, you might notice sensations that go all the way down into your genitals! It's totally yummy! You can download the entire meditation at this link (active at the time of publication): https://powerofpleasure.com/chocogasm-meditation/.

Slowing down foreplay is so important for women because a woman's sexual arousal is quite different than that of a man. If you touch a man's cock, he will often become aroused and be ready for sex within a short period of time. This is NOT true for women.

As Sheri Winston teaches in her book *Women's Anatomy of Arousal*, (Mango Garden Press, 2010), an excellent resource that I recommend that all my clients read, women have an extensive network of erectile tissue in our bodies, including the clitoris (head, shaft, and clitoral legs), vestibular bulbs, and the urethral and perineal sponges. But unlike men, most of our erectile tissue (e.g., genitals) is on the inside of our body except for our nipples, which need to be warmed up before being overly stimulated. Even our clitoris is covered by a hood! I like to analogize women's arousal to a cake being baked in the oven. We "cook" from the outside in, slowly and on a low temperature, and the inner part of our cake is the last thing to be ready.[23]

My general rule of thumb is that a woman is not ready for any type of penetration, be it finger or cock, until she is literally begging for it. And when you get to that point, your pussy will actually pull your partner's finger or cock inside of you like a vacuum cleaner. This is another way in which your body signals exactly what it wants. Mother Nature at her best!

Get Out of Your Head and Into Your Body

When you're in your head during sex, you reduce your ability to experience sensation. That keeps you from getting sufficiently

---

23 Sheri Winston, *Women's Anatomy of Arousal: Secret Maps to Buried Pleasure.* Kingston, NY: Mango Garden, 2010.

aroused. We all spend a lot of time in our heads, which is why the embodiment exercises that are available at myawakebody.com are so important. When you are in your head during sex, you simply cannot feel as much sensation in your body.

Here's a common scenario for a woman. You're enjoying some good foreplay and starting to feel really aroused. Maybe you're at a seven on a one to ten arousal scale. You start to realize that you are getting close to orgasm. You really want that orgasm and can't stop thinking about it.

Thinking about and wanting that orgasm takes you out of your body, significantly lowering your chances of reaching a climax. As backward as it may sound: the best way to have an orgasm if you're a woman is to not want to have one!

The Ins and Outs of Orgasm

Many women don't know that orgasm occurs from being both highly aroused and highly relaxed. In the simplest sense: orgasm is a release of energy, specifically, sexual energy. What happens when a body is in contraction? Energy gets stuck and cannot be released. The orgasmic release actually happens as a result of expanding and opening the body.

Here's another familiar scenario: You're pretty high on the arousal scale and feeling close to orgasm. The tension is building and you start clenching your butt and legs. At the same time, you start holding your breath. But nothing happens. The release doesn't come, and you're left with the female equivalent of "blue balls."

There is a simple reason the orgasm didn't happen: contracting the body and holding one's breath traps the sexual energy in the genitals, and then it can't be released. The energy literally has no place to go. The remedy for this is to allow breath, sound, and movement to move through your body as your arousal builds.

Breath, sound, and movement are the fuel that feeds the fire of your sexual energy and moves it around your body. In my work with women, we spend a lot of time learning various exercises to connect with sexual energy and move it around the body through these avenues.

As the sexual energy moves around the body, we start to feel more intense sensations. We continue to feel more sensation and we start to become aroused. With more sensation and more arousal, we have more energy to move around the body. Taking deep breaths into the belly and relaxing the butt muscles, we start to move the body freely, especially the hips. We feel the arousal continue to build and allow ourselves to make some noise.

It's worth repeating this phrase coined by Joseph Kramer, "The more you breathe, the more you feel." This is true on many levels. The deeper you breathe, the more oxygen you bring into your body. This oxygen is delivered to capillaries and nerve cells, which in turn helps to awaken more physical sensation in your body. This is the reason why you may feel warmth or tingling sensations when you are doing a breathing exercise. Deep breathing also activates the vagus nerve, which is connected to all of our organs, including our skin. Breathing also helps us to feel more of our emotions. It's not at all uncommon to get quite emotional when we get into slow, deep breathing. When we are connected with our emotions, we are also more connected with our sexuality. Likewise, when we are more connected with our sexuality, we are more connected with our emotions. A closed heart usually means a closed pussy.

The Power of Touch

Let's turn our attention now to touch. It is the first of our senses that develops in utero, and as such, touch is the first language we learn. Soft, gentle touch releases oxytocin into the bloodstream, creating trust. That trust in turn reduces cortisol, the stress hormone. Research studies on touch demonstrate that it helps premature infants gain weight, increases compassion, fosters cooperation over competition, and even results in NBA Basketball teams winning more games. Touch can convey a myriad of emotional states: anger, fear, disgust, love, gratitude, sympathy, happiness, sadness.[24]

We think that the process of touching a partner is quite straightforward, but in fact, there is a whole relationship dynamic involved in touch. Betty Martin, a well-known sex educator, has created a whole body of work around touch. In her workshops, she teaches a process of giving and receiving touch that allows each partner to consider their boundaries, what they are willing to give, what they are willing to receive, how they want to be touched by their partner, and how they want to touch their partner.

---

24 "Hands on Research: The Science of Touch," 2010. https://greatergood. berkeley.edu.

Exercise: The Three Minute Game

In Betty Martin's Three Minute Game (adapted from the work of Harry Fadis), partners take turns asking each other two questions. "How would you like me to touch you for three minutes?" and "How would you like to touch me for three minutes?" These seemingly simple questions actually require a lot of communication. You assume four different roles in this game based on whether you are touching or your partner is touching and whether you are giving a gift of touch or receiving a gift of touch. Martin identifies four different roles:

- Serving or taking action for the benefit of others: Ask what your partner wants. Decide if you are willing to do that. Check in on your own boundaries. Ask yourself, "Can I give this with a full heart?" If "yes," do your best. If "no," negotiate with your partner.

- Accepting or receiving the benefit of the actions of others: This is about you and knowing what you want. Ask directly and specifically. Feel free to make adjustments or change your mind. Don't worry about your giver's experience. The giver also has to check in with their boundaries and be a full "yes."

- Taking action for your own benefit: Check in with your partner about their boundaries. Notice how you would like to touch them within their boundaries. Ask your partner, "May I (touch your arm)?" not, "Would you like me to (touch your arm)?" Focus on your own sensations in your hands. This touch is for your own pleasure, not to "give to them."

- Allowing others to take action while keeping your own boundaries: Get clear on your own boundaries. Ask yourself, "Is this a gift I can give with a full heart?" Make sure you are a full "yes." A "maybe" or hesitation means either you are a "no" and need to express that or you need more details and information until you are a full "yes."

Touching for Your Own Pleasure

In Martin's game, the role of "taking" contains a principle of touch that will completely change your experience of pleasure. The principle is touching for your own pleasure. The principle is a mindset shift, meaning you will start to look at the whole arena of touch from a different perspective than that to which you are accustomed.

Generally, when we touch our partners, we are not doing it for our own pleasure and sensation. You touch your partner the way you think they want to be touched. If you are really attuned to your partner, you might ask them for feedback about your touch and then make an adjustment based on their response. On the other hand, touching for your own pleasure means that you touch your partner in a way that feels really good to you, focusing specifically on the sensations in your hands. When you touch your partner in a way that brings you pleasure, your partner will experience more pleasure. It feels that much better for your partner. Your partner is turned on by the pleasure you are experiencing, which increases their own enjoyment of your touch, which increases your own turn-on, thus creating a pleasure circuit between the two of you.

We are typically pretty unconscious about the sensations in our hands, but our hands have more nerve endings than many other parts of our body and can experience a tremendous amount of pleasure. The following exercise will give you a feel for what it means to touch for your own pleasure.

Exercise: Touching for Your Own Pleasure

Find a wine glass and place it in front of you. Place a pillow on your lap. Sit back in a relaxed position and shut your eyes. Hold the wine glass in your hands while resting your arms on the pillow. Keeping your arms and hands in a relaxed position for this exercise is very important. For the next few minutes, explore the wine glass. Go really slow and notice all the nuances of the glass. Feel all of the parts of the wine glass; cup, rim, stem, base. Notice the textures of each of these areas. Now touch the wine glass with various parts of your hands (fingertips, nails, palms, back of hand, wrists). Notice the mixture of textures and sensations as you use different parts of your hand. Now slow your touch down even more and really notice the sensation in your hands.

Again, try touching the object with different parts of your hands in a very slow and deliberate way, focusing on the sensation in your hands. Notice any pleasure you get from feeling those sensations. Notice what gives you the most pleasurable sensations and go back to that stroke for a few minutes. Imagine that the wine glass is a favorite body part. Touch the wine glass sensually, as if you are making love to it. Notice other parts of your body that might also be experiencing sensation and pleasure.

Because the wine glass is an inanimate object that has no reaction to your touch, this exercise will begin to awaken the nerve endings in your hands. The more awake the nerve endings become, the more aware you will be of the sensations in general as well as the subtleties, such as temperature, softness, etc. The only pleasure that you can derive from this exercise is from the sensations you create in your hands. This is truly about touching for your own pleasure.

Next time you are with a partner, take what you learned from this exercise and touch them with your eyes closed. We can usually focus more on our own sensations when we close our eyes, at least in the beginning. Once you are really feeling your pleasure, open your eyes and continue touching your partner. Notice other sensations in your body as well as whether there is any arousal for either one of you.

You are Responsible for Your Arousal

Here's another mindset shift for you. Once you understand this, you will be well on the way to experiencing more pleasure. You, and only you, are responsible for your sexual arousal. This is especially true for women because our arousal patterns are constantly shifting. As mentioned in Chapter 11, a woman's arousal is linked to many factors. What turned you on yesterday might turn you off tomorrow, and what has you writhing with pleasure for twenty minutes might suddenly feel unpleasant. This is totally normal; it is a natural result of the fact that nerves get tired and need time to rest.

This is one of the biggest frustrations couples have with their sex life. Reacting that way makes sense if you approach sex as science rather than, as Nicole Daedone suggests, as an art form. If you believe that there's a specific recipe for your arousal, that if you have all the right ingredients, you can expect the same outcome each and every time, you will be frustrated when that doesn't happen. You may even begin to think that something is wrong or that you're broken. But if you look at engaging in sex and pleasure as an art form, as dynamic and changeable rather than static and predictable, everything changes. Sex becomes intriguing, a discovery process, rather than a destination or a desired "result," i.e., orgasm.

The truth is that the only person who knows what gives you pleasure is you, and the only time you can know what gives you pleasure is in the moment. I'm very aware of my body and sensations during sex. I know my arousal patterns and give my partner very concrete feedback. But even with this slow sex approach and conscious environment, my partner sometimes gets frustrated. For example, he may think that the way he's giving me oral sex should bring me to orgasm because it did the last five times. When it doesn't, he could start blaming himself, which could easily lead us down into a negative spiral. I help defuse the situation by taking responsibility for my own arousal. "Wow, I'm just not feeling that right now, but what would feel really great for me is for you to suck my nipples." The result: I get what I want and need, and he feels no blame.

Learning What You Want

It's hard, if not impossible, to tell your partner what you want if you don't understand your own arousal pattern. A wonderful partner, especially one who knows how, where, and when you like to be touched, can increase your arousal; however, it is not their responsibility to figure out your arousal pattern. This is really challenging for many women because a fairly universal problem in our sex lives is that we don't know what we want. We've been socialized to believe that "sex just happens," and with each new partner, we hope that they've got the requisite experience and skills. This is why Betty Martin's Three Minute Game can be so useful: it allows you to discover how you like to be touched. Knowing this, you become an active participant in the process of receiving pleasure, rather than a passive receiver who goes along with whatever your partner is doing or thinks you want.

It's best not to assume that your partner knows what turns you on. Nor should you assume that your partner has all the skills they need to give you pleasure. After all, no one teaches us to have sex. We learn from trial and error, by reading books, and by watching movies or porn. Very few people learn specific techniques and skills from qualified teachers, and as we talked about before, most men assume a woman's arousal is just like theirs. Touch her clitoris and nipples, and she's ready to go.

In my Master Lover Workshops,[25] we teach men specific skills and techniques to become better lovers. In a real-time setting, they learn how to be present and how to connect with their own sexual energy and with that of a woman. They learn how to initiate and escalate a sexual encounter. We also demonstrate techniques for sensual massage on a female model, including Yoni and G-spot massage. This information is really crucial to a man's sex education. Most men are fairly clueless and do not spend enough time on foreplay. They touch nipples and genitals far too soon, use too much pressure, and don't really know how to build up arousal in women.

Unfortunately, very few men get to have this type of hands-on education. As a result, many men have performance anxiety when trying to get a woman to come. It's a repetitive cycle that does not have a happy ending for either one of you. It doesn't have to be so! And the solution starts with you learning what you want so you can give him the feedback he needs. In general, men love to learn skills and techniques and understand our bodies better. It's in their nature to want to please a woman. But they need us to provide them with direction and feedback; otherwise, they are fumbling around in the dark.

The best way for you to know what you want is to get to know your own arousal pattern by creating a self-loving (masturbation) practice. And I'm not talking about a five-minutes-with-your-vibrator type of practice. There is nothing wrong with that from time to time when you need an orgasm or a good release. I'm talking about blocking out thirty to forty-five minutes to really

---

25 Visit this link to learn more: powerofpleasure.com

connect with your body and your pussy slowly and intentionally. This is one of the most potent ways to connect with your own life force energy and orgasmic potential. I always have a self-loving session before I start a new project as it helps to awaken my creative energy and allow ideas to flow from a place of intuition rather than from a rigid structure.

The idea of a self-loving practice might be uncomfortable for you; maybe it even brings up some shame. Masturbation shame is very common for women, especially if your sexual blueprint contains negative messages about sex or you have a lot of body shame. If this is an issue for you, acknowledge it and do the Sexual Blueprint and Body Talk exercises in Chapter 4. When you do the following self-loving practice, go slowly, follow the sensation, and go as far as you are comfortable. Focus your initial practice solely on feeling sensation on your arms, face, and neck. The next time you practice, you can include your legs and belly. Then you can move to your breasts and go from there. Take your time and focus on relaxing and enjoying the touch without any goal orientation.

Exercise: Self-Loving Practice

I teach a very thorough self-loving practice, including G-spot exploration, in my Empowered Woman's Guide to Orgasmic Bliss[26] online class. But here is my quick recipe for a self-loving practice:

- Set a time limit for yourself of thirty to forty-five minutes. This need not be a marathon, especially if it's going to become a regular part of your week. A daily practice will give you the most benefit, but three or four times a week is awesome.

- Set an intention for your practice that isn't goal-oriented. This is not about having an orgasm, but rather about experiencing sensation and pleasure.

- Have your toys and supplies handy (lube, coconut oil, vibrators, dildos, anal plugs, feathers, and other sensate objects, as well as wet wipes, towels, etc.).

- Spend the first five to ten minutes getting into your body by putting on some sexy music and starting to move. Remember to continue to breathe!

- Start touching yourself while you are warming up, possibly with some soft furry objects like a scarf or a feather. Make it sexy and do what feels good for you.

- When you feel warmed up, find a comfortable position in your special space and start touching yourself for your own pleasure. Touch all parts of your body while ignoring the genitals for a period of time. While breathing, focus on the sensations in other parts of your body. What gives you goosebumps; what creates heat?

- Once you're starting to feel somewhat aroused, turn your attention to your pussy. Again, touch your pussy for your own pleasure, exploring all the nooks and crannies in the labia. Don't just go for the clitoris; let that be the icing on the cake. Gently massage your labia, one lip at a time. Pull at them, run your fingers down

26 Learn more by visiting: https://powerofpleasure.com/orgasmic-bliss-program

them, tickle them. There are thousands of nerve endings in this area, take your time to explore them!

- If clitoral stimulation works for you, explore the clitoris, but try varying the pressure and touch, especially if you are used to only touching yourself one way. Explore vaginal stimulation as well with fingers, toys, vibrators, etc. Remember that the focus is not on orgasm but on exploring pleasure in your body and learning your own unique arousal patterns.

- Don't be laser focused as you move into genital stimulation. Periodically revisit your breasts, belly, neck, ass, arms, legs, and other places on your body that feel good so that you can disperse the energy to other pleasure centers.

Orgasms Don't Just Happen in Your Genitals

While orgasm need never be the goal, you can experience orgasms in many different parts of your body, not only your clitoris. This makes sense because an orgasm is a release of sexual energy that has built up in the body. You can create and feel sexual energy in many other parts of your body besides your genitals. You can have orgasms from nipple stimulation and from anal, cervical, or G-spot stimulation. I've experienced orgasms from having my neck, ears, and belly bitten and stimulated. You can also experience energy orgasms from intense breath work with no physical contact or stimulation. In fact, there are numerous reports of paraplegics who have lost genital sensation experiencing orgasms in other body parts, including a thumb.

When we talk about reaching your orgasmic potential, the most powerful orgasms that you can experience are not from clitoral stimulation. A clitoral orgasm is an "outgasm," meaning that the energy goes out of your body, usually in a short burst that only lasts seven to ten seconds. On the other hand, a vaginal, G-spot, or cervical climax is an "ingasm," meaning the orgasmic energy flows into the body. The actual experience of a vaginal orgasm is much different than a clitoral orgasm. Rather than experiencing a short burst of energy and release, it may feel more like a big surge of energy you ride like a wave.

The sensations are different because there are two different sets of major nerves that are involved. The nerve involved in a clitoral orgasm is the pudendal nerve, which connects to your genitals, including the clitoris and the urethral sponge (G-spot). However, the pelvic nerve connects to other parts of your body, including the uterus, bladder, anus, and deep layers of the pelvic floor. Stimulating the organs connected to the pelvic nerve (the anus, cervix/uterus, and vaginal walls) creates sensations that come from much deeper in the body. They involve movement of the uterus, which give us the "OMG, what the f*** was that?!" sensation that often occurs from deep penetrative sex. The sensations are earth-shattering as you move into a different level of consciousness. Using the tools of breath, sound, and movement, this type of orgasm can be sustained for long periods of time, becoming increasingly intense with continued stimulation.

The vagus nerve is also involved in the orgasmic response. The vagus nerve is a cranial nerve that touches every organ system, including the skin, and is involved in both the sympathetic and parasympathetic nervous systems. When this nerve is activated by intense breathing and sounding, it stimulates the whole body, which creates the experience of whole body orgasms. Vagus nerve stimulation is responsible for non-genital orgasms such as nipple and energy orgasms, and it is the reason why someone who is paraplegic can have a thumb orgasm.

Anal Pleasure

Finally, let's talk about your often-neglected, frequently shamed anus, which can give you immense pleasure. I know that many of us shy away from anal play because it feels dirty and embarrassing and we believe anal penetration will hurt. I do not hold myself out as the queen of anal play, but I do want you to know the truth versus fiction.

HERE ARE SOME FACTS ABOUT ANAL PLAY:

- Your anus has thousands of nerve endings with immense pleasure potential.

- Many nerve endings are right around your butthole. Gently running a finger around the opening can feel amazing and is a great first step.

- Poop is not usually a problem as stool is not stored in the rectum. It's stored deeper in the digestive tract. You can always use latex gloves or do a gentle saline enema beforehand.

- Your G-spot can be activated through anal play with fingers, a toy, or a cock.

- Using lots of lubrication and going very slowly with just one finger is the best way to start.

- The more relaxed you are, especially your butt, the more enjoyable the experience. Deep breathing into your pelvis is quite helpful.

- Penetrative anal orgasms can be mind-blowing, especially if combined with a vaginal orgasm, because the pelvic and pudendal nerves are both involved.

Anal stimulation is great for women with tight pelvic floors. You can use a butt plug, which can be found in all different sizes, to help open up the anus, which will increase sensation in the vagina. I often recommend this for my vaginismus clients and for women who are experimenting with anal play for the first time.

It is perhaps fitting that we just talked about your butt since we're headed to the end of your sexual awakening journey. But what lies ahead of you are some real-life examples of what happens when you access your orgasmic life force energy and live an orgasmic life.

Chapter 14

· · · · · · · · · · · ·

LIVING AN ORGASMIC LIFE

· · · · · · · · · · · ·

Why is sexuality such a powerful doorway into personal growth and expansion? Why do I consider it a prerequisite to living an orgasmic life? Because our very existence and the continuation of our species depend on our sex drive. The biological mandate to copulate is at the very core of who and what we are. There is no energy more powerful than the ability and drive to create new life.

Sex is a Basic Human Need, Like Food and Shelter

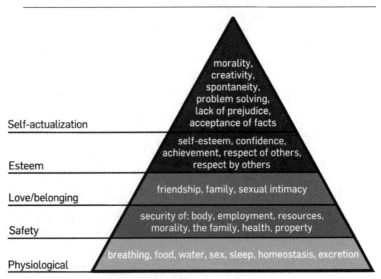

Maslow's hierarchy of needs

In Maslow's hierarchy of needs, sex is at the bottom of the pyramid, along with shelter, food, water, and sleep. It's interesting that sex is the only need in Maslow's model that shows up twice: at the base of the pyramid along with our physiological (survival) needs, and again on the third level, which he identifies as the need for love and belonging. From the perspective of Tantra, sexuality can propel us on our way toward reaching the apex of Maslow's pyramid, where we satisfy the highest need, self-actualization and self-transcendence. The sexual bliss we experience in Tantra comes from connecting our sexual energy with spiritual or divine energy to transcend our current mindset to a different state of consciousness. This transcendence brings on a sense of timelessness and the merging of yourself, your partner, and the universe. It's as if you disappear into each other and into a different realm, connecting with cosmic energy.

Transformation happens quickly through sexuality because this creative life force energy is so potent. I first came to the realization that sexuality has the power to transform every aspect of a person's life when I read Naomi Wolff's book, *Vagina*. Wolff's key premise is that a woman's vagina is the center of her creativity and personal power.[27] This perspective had a profound impact on me. Suddenly I understood why my life was changing at such a rapid-fire pace as I was becoming sexually alive and awake. The flow that I was clearly experiencing, of new doors opening at exactly the right time, creativity pouring out of me, and a deep sense of trust in the unknown, was my first experience of living an orgasmic life.

27 Naomi Wolff. *Vagina*. Ecco, 2012. Print.

A Sexual Woman is a
Creative Woman

Wolff links women's sexuality and their creativity by chronicling eighteenth and nineteenth century writers, painters, and artists such as Edith Wharton, Charlotte Bronte, Elizabeth Barrett Browning, and Gertrude Stein. Through their lives and work, each of these women expressed intense passion and gave birth to works of art that revealed their sexual nature. Wolff further makes her case by surveying over 16,000 women on Facebook about the connection between sexuality, self-confidence, self-love, and creativity. The results of the survey showed that, indeed, women do experience increased energy, creativity, self-expression, and self-confidence after having peak sexual experiences and transcendent orgasms.

A transcendent orgasm feels to me like an out-of-body experience so intense that I am not fully aware of my surroundings. It almost always results from G-spot or cervical stimulation and feels like waves of pleasure washing over me. I often experience many days of creativity after this type of orgasm. In fact, the five-page outline for this book practically wrote itself after a juicy self-loving session!

At a purely biological level, a woman who has frequent orgasms and is in touch with her sexual energy has higher dopamine levels than a woman who is sexually inactive or unfulfilled. This "feel good" chemical helps us stay focused, motivated, and energized. Dopamine also creates cravings and is highly addictive. When a woman is having great sex and the dopamine is flowing, she wants more and more sex to satisfy her dopamine cravings. The state of "bliss" and "oneness" many women experience from transcendent sex is largely due to opioids that are released during orgasm. Low dopamine levels contribute to a lack of ambition and are contributing factors in depression, loneliness, and a low libido.

The inherent power of sexual energy goes well beyond changes in brain chemistry. When we tap into our sexual centers—the uterus, ovaries, and vagina—we connect with our creative life force energy. The ability to create a new life is still magical and mysterious, even though we fully understand the science behind it and can even recreate it in a petri dish. And yet, there is another force at play when a sperm fertilizes an egg, a power that is bigger than us.

Sex Transmutation

This same power, our life force energy, which originates in the pelvic bowl, not only creates new human life; it is the root of our creative potential. Every invention, every new way of doing things, every innovation in business, manufacturing, and design is the product of human beings endowed with creativity. Every new work of art, new relationship, new idea, and new religion derives from the human capacity to create something new. The human creative potential is what sets us apart from the animal kingdom. Our drive to transform our lives, our surroundings, and our relationships makes us feel alive and keeps us going.

Research published in 2005 in the "Proceedings of the Royal Society" shows that creative people such as artists and poets are more sexual and have more sexual partners than the average adult. When we tap into our sexual energy, we open the doorway to our creativity. Our vision expands, we see new possibilities, and we are able to connect the flow of sexual energy to the flow of creative energy. Some of this emanates from physiological changes that take place in our bodies. Increased focus, improved clarity of vision, and vibrant energy are necessary for the creative process to unfold. I certainly feel this way when my creativity is flowing. It's as if I'm on fire, and words and ideas stream out effortlessly.

But this creative energy can also flow without the necessity of sexual activity as long as we are connected to the core of our sexuality. This is not "new age" thinking. In 1937, Napoleon Hill, author of the classic self-help book *Think and Grow Rich*, wrote about "sex transmutation," the ability to tap into the emotion of sex to get ahead in business and in life. Transmutation involves changing a state of being into another form. According to Hill, "It's an energy that can be directed into many channels. Anything you do can be electrifying and positive and profitable when it is infused with sex emotion. Transmuted sex energy can add warmth to your handshake, strength to your voice, attraction to your personality."[28] Tony Robbins, Meryl Streep, and Michael Jordan all transmute their sexual energy to create powerful performances that impact their audiences. My public speaking coach taught me to speak from my Yoni. When I do that, my whole demeanor changes. My posture is straighter, I feel more grounded, and my voice drops to a deeper, more authoritative resonance.

Quantum Physics and Sex

When a woman taps into her creative life force energy and is fully in her flow, she also can harness the quantum physics Law of Attraction popularized in *The Secret*, a bestselling self-help book written by Rhonda Byrne. Byrne claims that by using positive thinking and visualizations, you can change your life and manifest whatever you desire. A critical element of the Law of Attraction

---

28 Napoleon Hill, *Think and Grow Rich*. New York: Jeremy P. Tarcher/Penguin, 2005.

is that you can attract both positive and negative vibrations into your life and those magnetize other similar vibrations.[29]

We've all experienced or witnessed the Law of Attraction. Think about a time in your life when things were going your way, when opportunities were lining up, and when life felt effortless and you were "in the flow." You were on top of the world and the possibilities seemed limitless. Contrast this with a time when things weren't going your way, progress was slow, and life was a struggle. Your days were so peppered with disappointment that your outlook became pessimistic. From the perspective offered by the Law of Attraction, our circumstances don't "just happen" to us. Rather, we actually draw into our lives experiences that match our vibration—sometimes intentionally and sometimes without awareness. Either way, the Law of Attraction remains operational and essentially creates our reality. Said simply (and to quote the Bible), "We reap what we sow." My ex-husband is a prime example of how the Law of Attraction works when you have a pessimistic world-view. He is masterful at attracting challenging situations and people into his life and cannot comprehend how he enables that.

This universal law is highly relevant to sexuality—specifically, with respect to the process of reclaiming your sexual energy. When you connect to your sexual energy, your creativity awakens. The more you move your sexual energy and express your creativity, the more robust your life force becomes. The resulting vibration attracts even more creative energy. More and more, you experience positivity in all its forms. You may notice that you're walking with a bounce in your step. Friends may say, "You look different." Ideas, opportunities, and new relationships flow your way. Creative

---

29 Rhonda Byrne, *The Secret.* Atria Books, November 2006.

energy and sexual energy feed and amplify each other. Orgasmic life force energy transforms your whole life, which begins to flow in new, exciting directions.

You can help develop your creative potential by engaging in activities that are expressive in nature, something other than reading a book, watching TV, or surfing the Internet. These activate the right side of your brain, are more kinesthetic, and take you out of your head.

Exercise: Feed Your Creativity

This exercise is from Tami Lynn Kent's book, *Wild Creative: Igniting Your Passion and Potential in Work, Home, and Life.*

Find a quiet place, a pad of paper, and some colored markers.

1. Make a list of the various forms of creative expression you can imagine: photography, writing, singing, dancing, public speaking, gardening, cooking, drawing, expressing your style, decorating your home, playing music, sewing, crafting, painting, going to an art show or museum, sharing a new idea, designing a new project, making a playlist, shopping with friends, playing with your kids, having an adventure, trying a new sport, taking a creative class, doing something outside of your comfort zone, being intimate with yourself or a partner, or anything else that comes to mind.

2. Circle in yellow all the types of creative expression on your list that make you uncomfortable. Then circle in red anything that is associated with a negative feeling, such as discomfort or shame. Now circle in green your places of strength and ease. Notice the patterns that shape your creative range.

3. Now look at the bridges you can build between places of ease and those of discomfort. For example, if you feel awkward at parties but at ease when dancing alone in your house, try moving your body to music to free up your creative energy before you go out to a party. The creative energy that you access with ease can be put to good use broadening your creative range in the places you feel challenged.

4. Identify ways to leverage your strengths and use them to expand your creative range. Identify three key areas associated with challenges that you would like to reclaim and make a plan to do

so. Give yourself the permission and the means to embody the full range of your creative field.[30]

What did you notice in this exercise? Did anything surprise you? What bridges were you able to build? I have a lot of shame around singing and performing publicly because of some less than stellar performances I gave in summer camp musical theater productions during which I could not hit the notes or stay on key. But I love singing, so I pushed my edge and signed up for voice lessons and even agreed to sing in front of the class. I made sure to do some grounding and breathing exercises and connect with my Yoni. It was not nearly as painful as I had feared, and it helped me move through my shame.

30 Tami Lynn Kent, *Wild Creative: Igniting Your Passion and Potential in Work, Home, and Life*. Atria Books, 2014.

The Process of Transformation

Clients constantly ask, "How will I know when transformation happens?" It's a great question, but it does not have a clear-cut answer. Transformation often starts with a feeling that something is shifting inside. Many people describe it as an opening, as if a layer of your old self is being peeled away.

My transformation began with Tantra Man in New York. I started having regular sexual play. My body began the process of opening up. Within several months, I started to feel a shift of energy inside of me. The vision for my life started to come into focus. I had more energy and felt more fulfilled. I learned to listen to that little voice inside of me, even if the information I heard was not practical.

My first experience with G-spot (Sacred Spot) massage at Charles Muir's workshop was catalytic. I cried and mourned my marriage. I raged at Boston Man for all the lies and the times he'd mistreated and disappointed me. I screamed at the many doctors who had done painful medical procedures to treat my UTIs. On the other side of all of that pain and agony, I found pure bliss as sensations washed over my body and orgasmic energy began to flow. I left that workshop with a new understanding of my sexuality as a resource that was both magical and powerful. Little did I know where the path would lead and the magnitude of the impact this discovery would have on my entire life.

This experience is pretty commonplace for my clients when they start to awaken their sexuality.

Making a Career Change: Nora's Story

The email landed in my inbox two days before our Tuesday appointment. It was short and to the point, just like Nora. "Xanet,

I have big news to share with you." My mind went into overdrive thinking about all the possibilities. Had she met someone? Had something happened with her parents? Her job? Her house? I knew she had just returned home after a week-long retreat in Thailand and was curious to hear her news.

The minute she walked into my office, I knew something had changed. Instead of the usual fast-talking Nora exuding intense energy, the woman on my couch wore a look of deep serenity. Her face was soft and aglow, her eyes bright and sparkling.

"Something shifted inside of me during my retreat," she said. "I saw clearly that I needed to leave my company and do something else with my life. I've negotiated a year leave of absence to pursue my dream of starting my own clothing line."

"Wow," I said, "That's amazing. What happened on your retreat? Tell me all about the program." She laughed. "The first session did not resonate with me at all, so I decided to simply play and relax, just as you suggested. I spent the week drawing, meditating, and taking long walks. I got lots of massages, acupuncture, and Reiki sessions. I had some truly great orgasms from my self-loving practice. I began journaling and envisioning what this new life would look like. By the time I got on the plane to fly home, I had set up a meeting with my supervisor to discuss my plans."

Nora and I had talked many times about how unhappy she was in her job. She felt completely stuck in every aspect of her life at that time. Her relationships suffered, her family life fell into a slump, and she rarely felt her natural joy. She was not connected with her sexuality at all. We'd been working together for nine months to get her in touch with her feminine power when she decided to go on retreat to access her creativity, to give herself time and space to feel what was going on in her body, and to connect with her true desires. By the time the retreat drew to a close, she truly believed the universe would support her to fulfill her dream.

Intuition: The Greatest Gift of All

One of the key elements that drives transformation and the ability to live an orgasmic life is connecting with your intuition. Intuition is our brain's ability to draw on internal and external cues in making rapid, in-the-moment decisions—an important skill, particularly in high stress situations. Often occurring outside of our conscious awareness, intuition relies on our brain's ability to instantaneously evaluate both internal and external cues and make a decision based on what appears to be pure instinct.

PROVING INTUITION EXISTS

Researchers have struggled for years to prove that intuition exists and to find a way to scientifically measure it. A major breakthrough occurred in 2016. Researchers in Wales designed an experiment in which participants were exposed to emotional images outside conscious awareness as they attempted to make accurate decisions. The results of the study demonstrated that even when people were unaware of the images, they were still able to use information from the images to make more confident and accurate decisions. Two other findings were significant. Intuition improved over time, showing that it is a learned skill that can be strengthened with repeated use. The researchers also found physiological changes in the skin conductance of the subjects. Japanese researchers were able to conclude through brain imaging studies that intuition lies in the basal ganglia, a hub for learning and automatic behaviors.

How often do you have a gut feeling about some decision that you need to make? When you have that feeling, do you tend to listen to it or ignore it? There is a belief that women are highly intuitive and make decisions based on their intuition. The scientific research on this issue is inconclusive, although certain studies do show that the way the brain connects to different hemispheres differs in men and women. The authors of this study posit that these differences result in women being better able to integrate the intuitive right-brain hemisphere with the analytical left-brain hemisphere.

My own take on this is that it's not so much a function of the anatomical and neurobiological differences between men and women as how much of the right brain we women can access by tapping into our feminine energy. I have seen very analytical women who hold lots of masculine power and are unable to connect with their intuition. Conversely, highly intuitive men are typically able to access more of their feminine energy.

Women's intuition is often shut down due to forces outside of ourselves. Being told, "Don't get so emotional!" blocks our feeling, intuitive side. We are conditioned to rely on data, facts, and the judgments of others, even when our gut is telling us something else. There are often consequences from not listening to our intuition.

My worst financial investment came from not listening to my intuition and instead relying on data and logic. In 2006, the theater show *Dirty Dancing* was a major hit in London, and I was being courted to be one of the New York producers for a national ten-city tour. When I saw the show in London, I was so bored and unimpressed that I wanted to leave at intermission. They had basically taken the movie and put it on stage, word for word. That does not make for good or interesting theater. Yet audiences were eating it up, and the profits from the London show were tremendous. How could this not be a huge hit in the United States? I did not listen to my intuition and subsequently lost $1.5 million of investors' money, including $50,000 of my own. Ouch!

When I started to awaken sexually, I began really following my intuition and my life changed drastically. My second heart and second brain in my vagina were talking very loudly, and this time I was listening. To my surprise, the messages that I was receiving came not from my head, but from within my body.

While some people are born more intuitive than others, we all have intuitive abilities. Think about your intuition as a muscle that can be strengthened when you exercise it. Intuition happens in the body, so the more connected to and aware of your body you are, the more easily you are able to contact your intuition. This is why sexual awakening also activates your intuition.

Exercise: Cultivating Your Intuition by Learning Your "Yes" and "No"

In this practice, you are going to start listening to your body. Once you begin to heed the "yes" or "no" from your body, you will find it easier to make decisions that are right for you. Everyone's body speaks in its own language. Your job is to become familiar with how your body talks to you. This critical skill will give you greater access to your intuition.

1. Sit upright with your feet on the floor, close your eyes, and take a few deep breaths. Feel your body making contact with the chair. Allow yourself to completely relax. Notice any sensations you feel in or on your body.

2. Visualize your favorite food. Choose a food that makes your mouth water when you think about it. It could be chocolate, a steak, or sushi; whatever you like best.

3. Imagine that this food is right under your nose so you can really smell it. Remember its taste. Notice the flavors and textures.

4. Visualize putting this piece of food in your mouth. Notice its taste. Is it salty? Sweet? Both? Can you feel your salivary glands kicking in? Notice how the texture changes as you chew.

5. Move your focus to your body and scan it from head to toe. How do you feel? Are you open and relaxed? What part of your body is feeling sensations? When I do this with dark chocolate, my chest feels open, my belly is warm, and my pelvis is relaxed. I feel a comfort in my body. I recognize this as my body saying "yes." Notice where your body feels this "yes." It could be anywhere in

your body. You might even notice a color or a sound that goes along with this "yes."

6. Stand up, open your eyes, and shake your body.

7. Lie down again, close your eyes, and take a few breaths. Now we are going to visualize the opposite. Conjure up a food you absolutely detest. It could be eggplant, avocado, fish, or cilantro. Choose a food that makes you cringe and that puts a look of disgust on your face.

8. Imagine that the food is right under your nose so you can really smell it. Remember its taste. Notice its flavors and textures.

9. Visualize putting this piece of food in your mouth. Notice its taste. Is it salty? Sweet? Bitter? Notice how the texture changes as you chew.

10. Now move your focus to your body and scan it from head to toe. What part of your body feels sensations this time? When I think about drinking root beer, my throat closes up and my belly gets tight. I even feel a bit nauseous. I recognize this as my body saying "no." Notice where your body feels this "no." It could be anywhere.

11. You may find that you have to do this exercise several times before your "yes" and "no" become totally clear. Once you can hear your "yes" and "no" clearly, notice what happens in your body when you make decisions. Start with easy ones like, "What would I like to eat from the restaurant menu?" Ultimately, you can tap into your "yes" and "no" to make life-changing decisions.

Looking back, I realize that I have always had strong intuitive abilities, but my logical lawyerly left brain frequently dismissed those feelings, especially if they went against the grain. I started living an orgasmic life on the day that I decided to completely trust my intuition.

It was December 10, 2012, and I was sitting in my studio apartment in San Francisco. The previous year had been a whirlwind driven by my need for a change. I had left my home in New York City and resigned from a secure job. I was unemployed and unclear on my next step. When I was offered a position as vice president of business development for a San Francisco media organization, I jumped at the opportunity. Shortly after my arrival, I realized the company was in dire straits. Within two months, we were in merger talks. Come October, I was out of a job.

With an impressive resume, I imagined it would be easy to find another position. But I felt drained of my energy at the mere thought of taking a full-time job. During job interviews, my stomach and chest would get tight. I dismissed this crucial signal from my body as anxiety about being single and unemployed.

Nonetheless, I powered through interview after interview despite a tremendous amount of stress. I was scheduled for a final interview with a prestigious health care foundation in San Francisco. The recruiter told me I was their top candidate; the salary and benefits were impressive. The day before the interview, I felt queasy and had the runs all day long. Was I coming down with a bug? At 7 p.m. that night, I received word that my mother had died of Alzheimer's disease, just two days short of her ninety-fourth birthday.

I'd known Mom was on her deathbed for months, but the reality of her passing completely overwhelmed me. I cancelled the interview and told the recruiter I would get back in touch after my mother's funeral. But I never called her back. Death has a way of forcing you to reevaluate your priorities. As sad as I was about Mom's passing, I felt a huge weight come off my shoulders. I would have a small inheritance and could take a reprieve from working full-time for a year. I was grateful for the opportunity to examine what I wanted to do with the rest of my life. The answer was obvious…follow my intuition.

When we live an orgasmic life and are constantly in the flow, we experience transformation in many different aspects of our life: money, career, relationship status, and health and wellness. I could easily fill a book with stories of how my clients' lives have been radically transformed in each of these areas. Instead, I'm going to share the experiences of just three of my clients, and then we will turn our attention to helping you live an orgasmic life.

Making a Life-Changing Decision to Be a Single Mom: Lara's Story

Lara, a thirty-five-year-old single woman, was referred by a pelvic floor therapist. She was having pain with orgasms as a result of a medical procedure she'd had in her twenties. The physical therapy was helpful to a point, but Lara still had unresolved pain that did not appear to be physiological. After working together for a few sessions, it became clear that the trauma from the medical procedure was still held in her vagina. She was anxious and afraid that the condition would come back. She feared never being able to experience a pain-free orgasm again. As a result, she disassociated from her body during sex and physical sensations had become obscure and difficult to feel.

Initially, we focused on releasing the pent-up emotions related to the trauma. I showed her how to relax her pelvic floor during orgasms. She made rapid progress and began to resolve her sexual issues. Within a few months, she was enjoying sex.

In addition to her sexual issues, Lara had a hard time feeling her emotions. This is not uncommon. Blunted physical sensations and flat emotions often go hand in hand and make it difficult to make decisions. She found it hard to say "no," which left her little downtime for herself. Lara also hated her looks and felt uncomfortable in her body. She was certain that her skills in the tech world did not measure up to the exacting standards she had set for herself. As with many of my clients, once we did the initial work on her sexuality, Lara was able to address these other aspects of her life with greater clarity. Like so many men and women who reclaim their sexuality, she discovered powerful resources in her sexuality. She learned how to listen to her body and connect with her intuition. Lara became very clear on her desires and realized she wanted to be a mother, with or without a partner. She found a sperm donor and was pregnant in a matter of months. She found a better paying job with great maternity benefits. Shortly after giving birth, she met a man who eventually became her partner and her child's father.

When Sex and Creativity Flow, So Does the Money: Brant's Story

Brant was twenty-five years old when he came to see me. A tall, well-built Asian man, he had open wounds from a broken engagement. He carried a tremendous amount of shame around his sexuality—so much so that it was palpable. He could barely look into my eyes when I commented on his beautiful body. To help him connect with his sexual energy, I suggested we play a game and pretend to be wild animals in the jungle. We got down all fours and started to sniff and paw at each other. Initially, Brant was hesitant to touch me. But once we began to connect, he unleashed a ferocious inner lion, jumped on my back, and tackled me. Then he simulated taking me sexually, with clothes on of course. He had started down the road of transformation and progressed quickly through my coaching program.

Brant was also in flux as far as his career as a fitness professional. He worked part-time at a gym but was frustrated with the management and the structure of the fitness program. He was barely able to cover his expenses and could only afford to pay me the lowest amount on my sliding scale. By the time we completed our work together, he had been promoted to fitness manager and was working on starting his own personal fitness company. Today, Brant has a successful health and wellness company that offers nutritional counseling, fitness programs, and life coaching. He has become a mentor for at-risk youth, is a leader in the men's movement, and is completing his training as a sex and intimacy coach. When he reached a solid footing financially, he paid it forward and donated to my scholarship fund for clients in need.

Reinventing Herself in Her Sixties: Darleen's Story

I met Darleen at a Good Vibrations workshop. Her initial complaints—low libido and challenges with orgasm—were not surprising given that she was stuck in a sexless, loveless marriage that was draining her life force. She was anxious, depressed, physically depleted, and miserable in her job. She went to the gym for refuge and to feed her exercise addiction. She wanted desperately to leave her marriage but wasn't willing to give up the financial security. To complicate matters, she was having an ongoing affair that she'd led her husband to believe was over.

After a few months of sessions, Darleen became orgasmic, and even experienced a G-spot orgasm for the first time. Having tapped into the well of her sexuality, she easily made other changes. She took early retirement, left her husband, and went back to her roots as a therapist to pursue a career in grief counseling. She ended the hopeless affair and began a new dating life in her sixties. Darleen's body language reflected her transformation; she looked relaxed and open. Having let go of her exercise addiction and settled into a healthy weight, she began to fully enjoy her newfound freedom.

As you can see, when people get in touch with their sexual energy, they often make big changes in their lives, often in areas they weren't fully aware they wanted to change. This is the process of transformation. Once things begin to shift in one part of your life, that energy creates openings in other parts of your life as well.

Your Story Next

Living an orgasmic life means embracing all that life has to offer with a minimum of judgment. Being in the flow means trusting that there are lessons for us to learn in our joy and in our despair. Transformation is not a linear process. There are peaks and valleys, expansions and contractions, and patterns that will surely repeat themselves.

I've shared my story of transformation, as well as those of many of my clients. Now it's your turn to create your own story. Go back and look at what you wrote about in the Visioning Exercise in Chapter 8. What areas of your life would you like to change? Your relationship, sexuality, health, career, or financial security? Imagine how different your life could be once you connect to the creative and sexual energy that is your birthright. Every single one of my clients is just like you. They felt stuck in some part of their life; in a state of feeling broken and helpless, they didn't believe change was possible. Yet it was possible for them, and it is for you too. You can have great sex and successful relationships. Abundance, in every way, is yours for the asking. You can pursue your passion, whether it's a new career path or an extracurricular interest. Powerful transformation and personal growth are waiting for you. Go on, take the next step toward creating and living your orgasmic life.

Journaling
Prompts

Dear Reader,

The journey that you have embarked on towards living an orgasmic life requires self-awareness and reflection. To help you achieve some clarity, I am providing an opportunity for you to connect your own personal experiences with your challenges and desires through a series of journaling exercises related to each of the chapters. Journaling is one of the most powerful ways to process feelings and to reach new levels of awareness around your sexuality. The richness you will feel comes from focusing on the journey and not on the destination.

Chapter 2

·

Living a Life of Lies

·

Discuss what your sex life is like now and how you would like it
to change. What are the blocks that may be holding you back from
having the sex life you desire?

_____

_____

_____

_____

_____

_____

_____

_____

_____

_____

_____

_____

_____

_____

_____

_____

_____

_____

_____

CHAPTER 3

•

WOMEN ARE PROGRAMMED TO SAY "NO" TO SEX

•

Look at your own upbringing and the cultural messages that you received. How were you programmed to say "no" to sex? How do you see that programming showing up now in society?

_____

_____

_____

_____

_____

_____

_____

_____

_____

_____

_____

_____

_____

_____

_____

_____

_____

_____

_____

_____

Chapter 4

·

Shame: The Nastiest Five Letter Word in the Universe

·

How does body shame affect you?
What impact do you think it's had on your sexuality?

_____

_____

_____

_____

_____

_____

_____

_____

_____

_____

_____

_____

_____

_____

_____

_____

_____

Chapter 5

·

Sexual Abuse and Trauma

·

Every woman has had a sexual experience that did not meet her needs and expectations and left a bad taste in her mouth. Journal about that experience and notice feelings and emotions that are coming up. If you could hit the "replay" button, how would that experience change so that it had a positive outcome?

Chapter 6

•

The Body Remembers: Trauma and Physical Imprinting

•

List any injuries or physical wounds related to your sexuality.
This could range from a urinary tract infection to a hysterectomy.
Discuss how these wounds have impacted your sexuality.

_____

_____

_____

_____

_____

_____

_____

_____

_____

_____

_____

_____

_____

_____

_____

_____

_____

_____

_____

_____

_____

_____

_____

CHAPTER 7

•

BLOCKS TO INTIMACY

•

How has your attachment style (secure, anxious, avoidant, anxious-avoidant) affected your relationships with partners? How does it show up in dating or in long term relationships?

_____

_____

_____

_____

_____

_____

_____

_____

_____

_____

_____

_____

_____

_____

_____

_____

_____

_____

Chapter 8

·

Beginning the Journey of Sexual Healing and Awakening

·

Which of the four guiding principles to transform your sex life is most important for you right now?

○ Self-awareness and the courage to address your issues
○ Understanding and banishing your sexual shame
○ Accepting and loving your body, especially your vagina
○ Allowing yourself to fully experience pleasure

What are three actions that you can take to address it?

_____

_____

_____

_____

_____

_____

_____

_____

_____

_____

_____

CHAPTER 9

•

COMING HOME TO MY BODY AND WELCOMING PLEASURE

•

List five activities that give you pleasure and discuss how doing those activities makes you feel both emotionally and in your physical body.

_____

_____

_____

_____

_____

_____

_____

_____

_____

_____

_____

_____

_____

_____

_____

_____

_____

_____

Chapter 10

•

So What is Tantra Anyway?

•

If you've experienced sexual energy, describe what that feels like in your body. Under what circumstances did you experience it? If you believe you've never felt sexual energy, then how do you imagine it might feel? Is there an image of sexual energy that shows up for you (e.g., a spark of electricity?).

_____

_____

_____

_____

_____

_____

_____

_____

_____

_____

_____

_____

_____

_____

_____

_____

CHAPTER 11

·

HOW TO REIGNITE YOUR SHRINKING LIBIDO

·

Based on the themes we talked about in this chapter, what is the one most powerful action you can take now to increase your desire? Why did you choose this one?

_____

_____

_____

_____

_____

_____

_____

_____

_____

_____

_____

_____

_____

_____

_____

_____

_____

_____

_____

_____

_____

Chapter 12

·

Sexual Polarity: What Most Women Crave

·

Do you consider yourself to hold more feminine or masculine
energy and if so how does that manifest itself? Does sexual polarity
exist in your intimate relationships? What type of energy are you
typically attracted to and why?

_____

_____

_____

_____

_____

_____

_____

_____

_____

_____

_____

_____

_____

_____

_____

_____

_____

_____

_____

CHAPTER 13

•

REALIZING YOUR PLEASURE POTENTIAL

•

If you were to give your partner a guide to your very own night of receiving pleasure, what would that look like? This includes not only pleasure on your body, but also awakening your other senses.

_____

_____

_____

_____

_____

_____

_____

_____

_____

_____

_____

_____

_____

_____

_____

_____

_____

_____

_____

Chapter 14

·

Living an Orgasmic Life

·

How has your intuition impacted your life in a positive way?
Listening to your intuition, what words or phrases arise when you
consider what would need to change for you to live your life in a
more orgasmic flow?

_____

_____

_____

_____

_____

_____

_____

_____

_____

_____

_____

_____

_____

_____

_____

_____

Acknowledgments

In July of 2014, only one year after starting The Power of Pleasure, I sat down to write an outline of a book about my life journey. In reality, the outline wrote itself, and two hours later, I had a fairly comprehensive and detailed outline for this book. There was only one problem. I did not have sufficient experience, knowledge, training or clients to be able to write anything more than the personal sections of the book. So it sat in my computer for a few more years until 2016, when I created an end-of-year goal to complete the first draft of the book.

I'm still not sure I would be writing this acknowledgment had I not had the great fortune to meet Geralyn Gendreau at a mutual friend's house. A brilliant developmental editor, she helped me shape the book, taught me how to be a better and more interesting writer, and was a constant presence and unfailing cheerleader.

My dear friend and mentor Lokita Carter was pivotal in the initial editing process and helped me weave the thread of "living an orgasmic life" into every chapter of the book. Tantra comes in many forms! My colleague Jess Devries is an ace editor whose great questions and enthusiastic sidebar comments still bring a smile to my face. Huge appreciation to my Beta Readers, Lesli Doares, Simon Berkowitz, and Denise Ravizza, who gave me great feedback.

I was on the way to self-publishing until I met Lee Constantine from Publishizer.com, a crowdsourced funding platform that matches authors with publishers. Without his constant emails, phone calls, reminders, nudges, and cheerleading, I would never have gone the distance with my initial pre-sales launch, which ended up selling over 600 books and landed me a publishing deal.

Huge thanks to all of my dedicated readers who have waited so patiently for this book to come out!

I am extremely grateful for all the support from the folks at Mango Publishing: Brenda Knight, my incredibly energetic, brilliant, and astute editor, who has guided me through this process and constantly pushes me to get my work out in the public sphere; the marketing team of Michelle Lewy, Hannah Paulsen, and Ashley Blake; and amazing cover and design work by Morgane Leoni. And of course, thanks to CEO Chris McKenney, who was willing to take the risk.

I would be nowhere without my friends and family, especially my two boys, Marshall and Eddie, who have stood by my side, put up with Mom's crazy ideas, and continue to fill me with love.

References

Anand, Margot. *The Art of Everyday Ecstasy: The Seven Tantric Keys for Bringing Passion, Spirit and Joy into Every Part of Your Life* (Harmony 1999)

Anand, Margot. *The Art of Sexual Ecstasy: The Path of Sacred Sexuality for Western Lovers* (Jeremy P. Tarcher Inc., 1989)

Anand, Margot. *The Art of Sexual Magic: Cultivating Sexual Energy to Transform Your Life* (TarcherPerigree 1996)

Bahadur, Nina. "Women Want More Sex, Survey Says", huffingtonpost.com, 9/12/2015, https://www.huffingtonpost.com/entry/how-women-really-feel-about-sex-survey_us_55f83bdde4b09ecde1d9b5e6

Bergner, Daniel. *What Do Women Want? Adventures in the Science of Female Desire.* Harper Collins, 2014. Print. [pp. 94 and 163]

Blank, Joani. *Femalia.* Down There Press, 1993. Print. [p. 50]

Byrne, Rhonda. *The Secret.* Atria Books, November 2006. Print. [p. 201]

Charles, Amara. *The Sexual Practices of Quodoushka: Teachings from the Nagual Tradition.* Destiny Books, 2011. Print. [p. 50]

Chrystal, Paul. *In Bed with the Ancient Greeks: Sex & Sexuality in Ancient Greece.* Amberly Publishing, 2016. Print. [p. 32]

Daedone, Nicole. *Slow Sex.* Grand Central Life & Style, 2012. Print. [p. 176]

David Deida. *The Way of the Superior Man.* © 1997, 2004, 2017. Excerpted with permission of publisher, Sounds True, Inc.

Fisher, Helen. *Why We Love: The Nature and Chemistry of Romantic Love*. Henry Holt & Co., 2004. Print. [p. 162]

Glamour.com. "How Many Minutes Sex and Foreplay Really Last," Glamour Magazine, 2008. https://www.glamour.com/story/how-many-minutes-sex-and-forep. [p. 151]

Hands on Research: The Science of Touch: 2010 <www.greatergoodberkeley.edu> [p. 184]

Hebenick, Debby et al. *Sexual Behaviors, Relationships, and Perceived Health Status Among Adult Women in the United States: Results from a National Probability Sample*. The Journal of Sexual Medicine, Volume 7, 277–290, 2010

Hill, Napoleon. *Think and Grow Rich*. TarcherPerigree, 1937. Revised 2005. Print. [p. 201]

Hirschman, Celeste and Danielle Harel. *Making Love Real*. Somatica Press, 2015. Print. [p. 157]

Judith, Anodea. *Wheels of Life: A Journey Through the Chakras*. © 1999 Llewellyn Worldwide, Ltd., 2143 Wooddale Drive, Woodbury, MN 55125. All rights reserved, used by permission. [p. 130]

Kent, Tami Lynn. *Wild Creative: Igniting Your Passion and Potential in Work, Home, and Life*. Atria Books, 2014. Print. [pp. 203-204] Exercise: Feed Your Creativity

Kinsey, Alfred C. *The Kinsey Reports*. Indiana University Press, Reprint Edition, May 22, 1988, originally published in 1948 & 1953. Print. [p. 22]

Koch, Christopher. *Intuition May Reveal Where Expertise Resides in the Brain*. 2015. https://www.scientificamerican.com/article/intuition-may-reveal-where-expertise-resides-in-the-brain/ [p. 207]

Levine, Amir and Rachel Heller. *Attached: The New Science of Adult Attachment and How it can Help You Find and Keep Love.* Tarcher/Penguin, 2010. Print. [p. 88]

Levine, Peter. *Waking the Tiger: Healing Trauma.* North Atlantic Books, 1997. Print. [p. 56, p. 60]

Lewis, Tanya. *How Men's Brains are Wired Differently Than Women's* scientificamerican.com, 2013. https://www.scientificamerican.com/article/how-mens-brains-are-wired-differently-than-women/ [p. 208]

Lufityanto, G., Donkin, C., & Pearson, J., *Measuring Intuition: Nonconscious Emotional Information Boosts Decision Accuracy and Confidence.* Psychological Science, 2016. DOI: 10.1177/0956797616629403

Morin, Jack. *The Erotic Mind.* Harper Collins, 1995. Print.

Padoux, Andre. *The Roots of Tantra.* State University of New York Press, 2001. Print. [p. 125]

Pailet, Xanet. *How the Feminist Movement Has Ruined our Sex Lives and What We Can Do to Fix It,* Elephant Journal, July 2014. https://www.elephantjournal.com/2014/07/how-the-feminist-movement-has-ruined-our-sex-lives-what-we-can-do-to-fix-it-xanet-pailet/ [p. 167]

Schnarch, David. *Passionate Marriage: Keeping Love and Intimacy Alive in Committed Relationships.* W.W. Norton & Co., Reprint Edition, 2009. Print. [p. 152]

Spar, Deborah. *Wonder Woman: Sex, Power and the Quest for Perfection.* Picador, 2014. Print. [p. 167] van der Kolk, Bessel. *The Body Keeps the Score: Brain, Mind and Body in the Healing of Trauma*. Penguin Books, Reprint Edition, Sept 2015. Print. [p. 70]

Veale, D., Miles, S., Bramley, S., Muir, G. and Hodsoll, J., *Am I normal? A systematic review and construction of nomograms for flaccid and erect penis length and circumference in up to 15,521 men.* BJU Int, 115: 978–986. 2014. DOI:10.1111/bju.13010

Winston, Sheri. Women's *Anatomy of Arousal*. Mango Garden Press, 2010. Print. [p. 180]

Wolff, Naomi. *Vagina*. Ecco, 2012. Print. [p. 199]

Exercises

- Awakening New Pleasure Pathways by Xanet Pailet
- Body Talk Exercise by Xanet Pailet
- Chakra Sounding Exercise from Charles Muir, Source Tantra
- Chocogasm Meditation by Xanet Pailet
- Create Your Vagina Timeline from Tami Lynn Kent's book, *Wild Feminine.* Atria Books, 2011
- Cultivating Your Intuition by Learning Your "Yes" and "No" by Xanet Pailet
- Feed Your Creativity from Tami Lynn Kent's book, *Wild Creative: Igniting Your Passion and Potential in Work, Home, and Life.* Atria Books, 2014
- Fun Ways to Find Your Sexy by Xanet Pailet
- Identifying Your Hottest Sexual Movie from *Making Love Real,* Celeste Hirschman and Danielle Harel
- Peak Sexual Experience Exercise from the Peak Sexual Experience Survey from Institute for Advanced Study of Human Sexuality
- Sacred Space Ritual: A Partner Practice used with permission from the Ecstatic Living Institute's "Timeless Loving™ Workshop"
- Self-Loving Practice by Xanet Pailet
- Sexual Blueprint Exercise by Xanet Pailet
- Subtle Energy Exercise by Xanet Pailet
- The Three Minute Game by Betty Martin (adapted from the work of Harry Fadis)
- Touching for Your Own Pleasure by Xanet Pailet
- Visioning Letter by Xanet Pailet
- The Yoni Talk from "The Love & Ecstasy Training (LET)®" shared with special permission by Margot Anand

Recommended Resources

Note: This section is hardly comprehensive. There are hundreds of books about sex out there, but these are the ones that I keep on my bookshelves. I also would refer you to Joan Price's comprehensive list of resources in her book, *The Ultimate Guide to Sex After 50*. I will continue to expand and update this list on powerofpleasure. com. Let this be a start of your own personal exploration.

Sexual trauma and abuse

Beyond Surviving: The Final Stage in Recovery from Sexual Abuse by Rachel Grant

Rachel Grant has numerous outstanding resources available on her website: rachelgrantcoaching.com— including podcasts, a very active and large Facebook group, "Survivors of Childhood Sexual Abuse," and group and individual support.

Healing Sex: A Mind-Body Approach to Healing Sexual Trauma by Stacey Haines (Cleis Press, 2007)

In an Unspoken Voice: How the Body Releases Trauma and Restores Goodness by Peter Levine (North Atlantic Books, 2010)

Overcoming Trauma through Yoga: Reclaiming Your Body by David Emerson & Elizabeth Hopper (North Atlantic Books, 2011)

The Body Keeps the Score: Brain, Mind, and Body in the Healing of Trauma by Boessel van der Kolk (Penguin Books, 2015 Reprint)

Waking The Tiger: Healing Trauma by Peter Levine (North Atlantic Books, 1997)

Recommended Trauma Therapies/Workshops

Somatic Experiencing: www.traumahealing.org for a list of certified practitioners in the US and internationally

EMDR International: https://emdria.site-ym.com/ for a list of certified EMDR practitioners in the US and internationally

Smart Body Smart Mind: www.irenelyon.com – a comprehensive online workshop for healing the nervous system with advanced SE practitioner Irene Lyons.

Woman's sexuality

Come as You Are: The Surprising New Science That Will Transform Your Sex Life by Emily Nagoski, PhD (Simon and Schuster, 2015)

Our Bodies Ourselves: A New Edition for a New Era by Boston Women's Health Collective (Touchstone, 2017)

Sex for One: The Joy of Selfloving by Betty Dodson, PhD (Harmony, 1996)

She Comes First: The Thinking Man's Guide to Pleasuring a Woman by Ian Kerner (William Morrow Paperbacks, 2009)

Vagina by Naomi Wolf (Virago Press, 2013)

Woman's Anatomy of Arousal: Secret Maps to Buried Treasure by Sheri Winston (Mango Garden Press 2009)

Recommended Workshops and Classes

The Empowered Woman's Guide to Orgasmic Bliss: Xanet Pailet, www.powerofpleasure.com

Body Talk Workshop: Betty Dodson, PhD, www.dodsonandross.com

Jade Pleasure: Layla Martin, www.laylamartin.com

The Yoni Temple Retreat: Ashley Apple, www.ashleyapple.com

Motherhood and sex

Mothering from Your Center: Tapping Your Body's Natural Energy for Pregnancy, Birth, and Parenting by Tami Lynn Kent (Atria Books, 2013).

Sexy Mamas: Keeping Your Sex Life Alive While Raising Kids by Cathy Winks (New World Library, 2004)

Menopause and sex

The Ultimate Guide to Sex After 50: How to Maintain—or Regain—a Spicy, Satisfying Sex Life by Joan Price (Cleis Press, 2014)

The Secret Pleasures of Menopause: A Guide to Creating Vibrant Health Through Pleasure by Christiane Northrup, MD (Hay House, 2009)

The Hormone Cure: Reclaim Balance, Sleep, and Sex Drive by Sarah Gottfried, MD (Scribner, 2014)

The Female Brain by Louanne Brizandine, MD, (Harmony 2007)

Tantric Sex and Menopause: Practices for Spiritual and Sexual Renewal by Diane Richardson (Destiny Books, 2018)

Sexual exploration for couples

Guide to Getting It On by Paul Joannides (Goofy Foot Press, 2013)

The Little Black Book of Sex Positions by Dan and Jennifer Bartichi (Skyhorse Publishing, 2013)

Science for Sexual Happiness: A Guide to Reclaiming Erotic Pleasures by Caffyn Jesse (Eros Spirit, 2016)

Succulent Sex Craft: Your Hands-On Guide to Erotic Play & Practice by Sheri Winston (Mango Garden, 2014)

There are a number of really fun and creative sex phone apps for couples:

- Pillow
- Kamasutra
- Kindu
- 69 Places
- Dirty Game—Hot Truth or Dare

Tantra

The Art of Sexual Ecstasy: The Path of Sacred Sexuality for Western Lovers by Margot Anand (Jeremy P. Tarcher, Inc, 1989)

The Art of Everyday Ecstasy: The Seven Tantric Keys for Bringing Passion, Spirit and Joy into Every Part of Your Life by Margot Anand (Harmony, 1999)

The Art of Sexual Magic: Cultivating Sexual Energy to Transform Your Life by Margot Anand (TarcherPerigree, 1996)

The Couples' Kama Sutra: The Guide to Deepening Your Intimacy with Incredible Sex by Elizabeth McGrath (Sonoma Press, 2016)

Tantric Sex for Women: A Guide for Lesbian, Bi, Hetero, and Solo Lovers by Christa Schulte (Krug & Schadenberg, 2005)

Urban Tantra: Sacred Sex for the Twenty-First Century by Barbara Carrellas (Celestial Arts, 2007)

Recommended Tantra Schools

Ecstatic Living Institute: www.ecstaticliving.com

Source School of Tantra Yoga: www.sourcetantra.com

Quodoshka: www.qoudoshka.org

Urban Tantra: www.barbaracarrellas.com

Sexuality workshops and recommended practitioners

Ecstatic Living Institute: In addition to offering Tantra workshops, ELI also offers sexuality workshops such as Ecstatic Lover (created by Xanet Pailet and Kai Wu), Ecstatic Touch, and Ecstatic Relationships. www.ecstaticliving.com

Human Awareness Institute offers sexuality workshops for individuals and couples. www.hai.org

Holistic Pelvic Care offers training and a list of approved practitioners. www.wildfeminine.com

Sexological Body Work offers a list of certified sexological bodyworkers in the US and Internationally.
www.sexologicalbodyworkers.org

Somatica Institute offers training in The Somatica® Method of Sex and Intimacy Coaching, Couples Workshops, and Individual Coaching by Certified Somatica coaches.
www.somaticainstitute.com

About the Author

Xanet Pailet is a recovered New York City health care lawyer who lived in a sexless marriage for over two decades. After experiencing her own sexual healing and awakening in 2011, she transformed her career path and is now a full-time sex and intimacy coach, writer, blogger, and teacher. She works with individuals and couples to empower them around their sexuality and strengthen relationship and intimacy skills. Xanet is particularly passionate about working with women, men, and couples who are sexually disconnected. Through her work and the many tools that she offers, she helps them reclaim their pleasure and transform their relationships and their lives.

Xanet is a certified Somatica Sex and Intimacy Coach, Sexological Body Worker, Holistic Pelvic Care Practitioner, and Tantra Educator. She is on the faculty of the Ecstatic Living Institute and The Somatica Institute and teaches regularly at Good Vibrations in San Francisco. She offers one-on-one coaching via Skype or in person in the Bay Area. She also offers online group coaching programs and speaks regularly at national and local conferences and events. She lives in beautiful and serene Marin County, CA. Connect with Xanet at powerofpleasure.com.

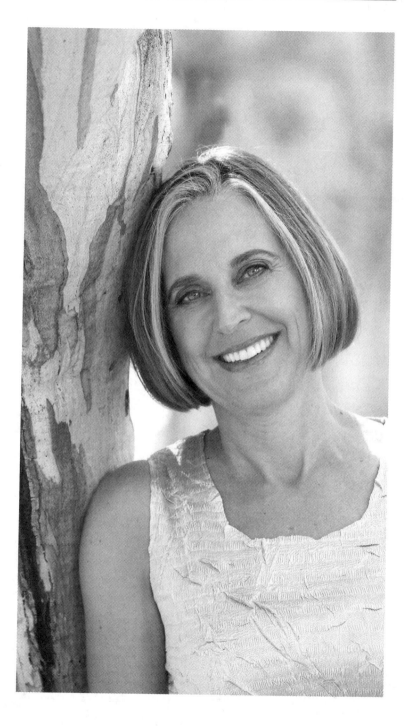